Calisthenics

Exercises for Beginners

The Complete Bodyweight Workouts to Build Strength, Control, and Confidence — No Equipment Needed

Lanzo K. Castillo

Copyright © 2025 by Lanzo K. Castillo

All rights reserved.

No part of this publication may be copied, reproduced, distributed, or transmitted in any form or by any means, including photocopying, recording, scanning, or by any electronic or mechanical methods, without the prior written permission of the author, except in the case of brief quotations for the purpose of reviews, references, or educational use.

This book is protected under international copyright laws. Unauthorized use, duplication, or distribution is strictly prohibited and may result in legal action.

Disclaimer:

The material in this book is provided for informational and educational purposes only. It is not intended as a substitute for medical advice, diagnosis, or treatment. Always consult with your physician or a qualified healthcare provider before beginning any exercise program, especially if you have any existing medical conditions or physical limitations.

The author and publisher disclaim any liability for injury, loss, or damage sustained directly or indirectly from the use of this material. Participation in any fitness program involves risk. The reader assumes full responsibility for their own safety and outcomes.

While every effort has been made to ensure the accuracy of the information contained in this book, the author makes no guarantees or warranties, express or implied, regarding the content, completeness, or results from following the program outlined within.

Table of contents

Introduction 4
    A Welcome to the Bodyweight Revolution 4
    Why Calisthenics Outperforms the Gym for Beginners 5
    What You'll Achieve with This Book 7
    How to Use This Guide 8

Chapter 1: The Fundamentals of Calisthenics 9
    What Is Calisthenics? Origins, Science, and Benefits 9
    Understanding Movement Planes and Muscle Chains 11
    Building a Foundation: Balance, Mobility, and Control 12
    Key Principles: Consistency, Form, and Progression 14

Chapter 2: Readiness & Recovery 16
    Self-Assessment: Where Do You Start? 16

Chapter 3: Mobility & Activation Essentials 22
    Mobility + Activation Exercises 22

Chapter 4: Core Foundation & Stability 31
    Core-Specific Exercises 31

Chapter 5: Push Mechanics for Beginners 42
    Push-Based Movements 42

Chapter 6: Pull Mechanics Without Equipment 51
    Pull-Based Movements 51

Chapter 7: Leg Strength & Lower Body Control 58
    Lower Body Exercises 58

Chapter 8: Balance, Coordination & Functional Flow 69
    Stability-Based Movements 69

Chapter 9: 28-Day Bodyweight Challenge 82

    Week 1: Foundation Phase... 83

    Week 2: Strength Integration 86

    Week 3: Progress & Precision 88

    Week 4: Control, Flow & Integration 90

Conclusion 93

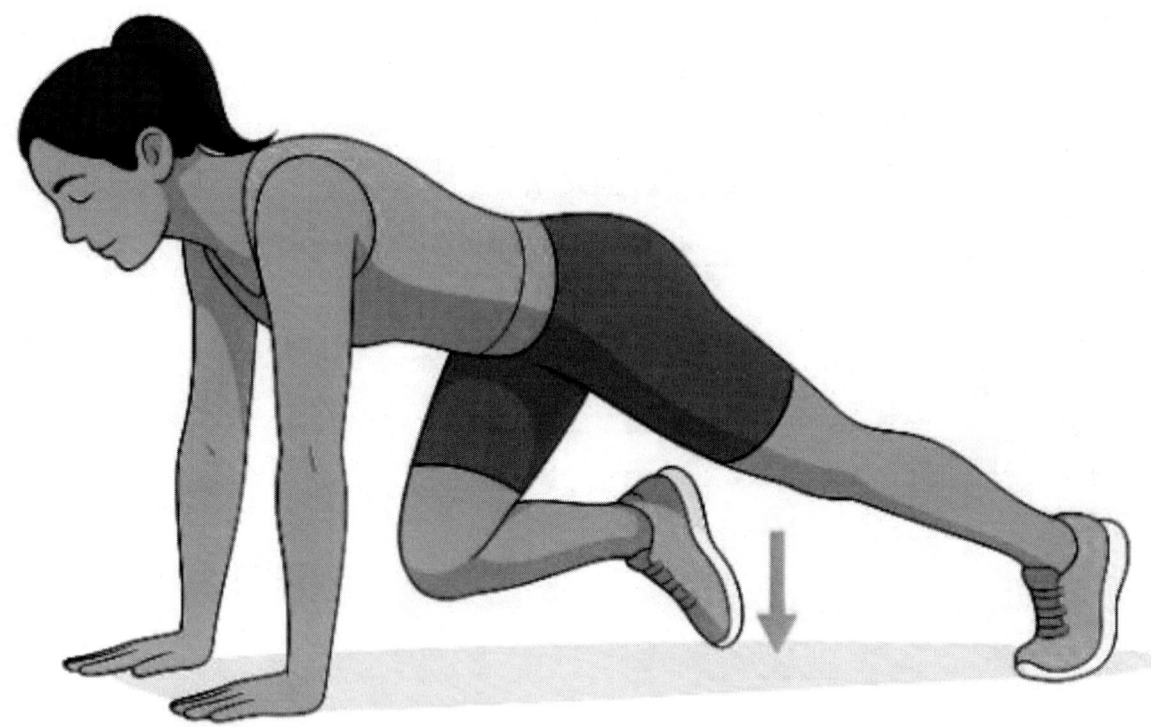

Introduction

A Welcome to the Bodyweight Revolution

I remember the first time I tried a push-up. I was flat on the floor within seconds — no strength, no control, no clue what I was doing. It was humbling, to say the least. I had always assumed that fitness meant lifting weights, using machines, or signing up for complicated programs. But here I was, struggling with one of the most basic bodyweight movements. And that's when it clicked: if I couldn't control my own body, what was I really training?

That moment started my journey into calisthenics — not the flashy, Instagram version, but the real process of learning how to move well, build strength from the inside out, and create consistency without relying on equipment or gyms.

If you're reading this, there's a good chance you're starting at the beginning — or starting over. And that's the smartest place to be. Calisthenics isn't about perfection or speed. It's about mastering the fundamentals that most people skip — the small details that create real, lasting results.

This book is built for you. Not for elite athletes or advanced practitioners. It's for the person who wants to move better, feel stronger, and stay consistent without needing a gym or a full hour every day. You'll learn how to train using nothing but your body, your breath, and your attention. And in doing so, you'll develop not just strength, but control — the kind that carries into everything else you do.

One of the biggest myths in fitness is that beginners need to "build a base" with machines or isolation movements before they can do bodyweight training. That's wrong. Calisthenics is the base. It teaches movement patterns, posture, balance, breathing, and coordination — all at once. The more you train this way, the more you realize how effective it is not just for fitness, but for life.

Every chapter in this book is structured with progression in mind. We'll start with mobility and activation, because your body has to move well before it can move hard. Then we'll build core control — the foundation for every push, pull, and squat. From there, we'll work through your upper and lower body in a smart, scalable way. No gimmicks, no endless reps — just the right movement, at the right time, for the right reason.

You'll also find a full 28-day program designed to keep you consistent and growing. You won't be left wondering how to put it all together — it's laid out for you, week by week. And by the end of it, you'll feel the difference. In your posture, in your endurance, in your strength, and in your confidence.

More importantly, you'll have built a habit. A way of training that doesn't depend on motivation or access to a gym. A system you can rely on, wherever you are, no matter what life throws at you.

That's what this book is really about — not just workouts, but ownership. Calisthenics gives you that. It brings everything back to you: your effort, your form, your discipline, your results.

So take your time. Read with intention. Train with purpose.

Why Calisthenics Outperforms the Gym for Beginners

Walk into any commercial gym and you'll see rows of machines, racks of weights, and people hopping from one station to the next. For a beginner, it's easy to feel lost — like fitness is some complex formula only a few understand. The truth? You don't need a gym to get strong. In fact, when you're just starting out, the gym can actually slow you down.

Calisthenics offers something the gym rarely does: ownership. You learn how to move *your* body, in *your* space, with *your* full attention. There's no machine locking you into position, no cables guiding the motion for you. Every movement in calisthenics demands engagement, awareness, and control — and that's exactly what builds real strength.

Let's break it down.

1. You Build Strength That Transfers to Real Life

Pushing your body off the floor, squatting your own weight, holding your core stable in space — these are functional skills. They train the muscles *and* the nervous system. The strength you develop with calisthenics carries over to everyday movement: climbing stairs, lifting groceries, improving posture, even reducing pain.

Machines isolate. Calisthenics integrates.

2. You Start with What You Already Have

No waiting for equipment. No travel time. No gym fees. All you need is your body and a bit of floor space. That means fewer barriers to entry — and no excuses. You can train anywhere: at home, in a park, or even in a hotel room. The accessibility of calisthenics removes friction, and that's one of the biggest reasons beginners stick with it.

3. You Develop Control, Not Just Muscle

In the gym, it's easy to chase numbers — more weight, more reps, more speed. But what happens when you never learned to move well in the first place? Calisthenics starts with movement quality. It teaches you how to stabilize, how to breathe, and how to feel when a rep is done right — not just when it's done.

And the irony? When you focus on control first, the results actually come faster — and they last longer.

4. You Reduce the Risk of Injury

Machines can create a false sense of stability. They guide the movement for you, often at the expense of joint awareness and core engagement. Calisthenics forces your body to stabilize from the inside out — which means you're not just moving weight, you're controlling it. That's the difference between training that builds resilience and training that breaks you down.

5. You Learn to Train, Not Just Exercise

There's a difference between working out and training. Working out is random — it burns calories, but not always with intention. Training is progressive. It's built on structure. It teaches you how to improve, not just sweat. Calisthenics helps beginners shift from chasing effort to building mastery — and that's where real transformation begins.

You don't need machines to get strong. You don't need mirrors to check your form. What you need is consistency, a plan, and a commitment to getting better each time you train. Calisthenics gives you all of that — and it starts with your very first rep.

What You'll Achieve with This Book

This book isn't a crash course or a 7-day shortcut. It's a system — one that helps you build strength, mobility, and control from the ground up. If you follow the structure, stay consistent, and treat each rep with intention, here's what you can expect to gain:

1. Functional Strength You Can Feel

You'll develop real, usable strength — not just in isolated muscles, but across your entire body. You'll notice it when you carry groceries, get off the floor, or move through your day with more ease and less strain. Every movement in this book is designed to connect muscles, not separate them.

2. Better Balance, Posture, and Joint Health

Calisthenics sharpens body awareness. You'll improve how you move, how you stand, and how you stabilize. If you've struggled with tight hips, stiff shoulders, or poor posture, you'll start to feel a difference within weeks. You won't just look stronger — you'll move like it.

3. Core Stability That Translates Into Everything

Forget endless crunches. You'll learn how to build a core that supports you in every movement — whether it's a push-up, a squat, or simply holding a plank with control. Strong core engagement is the secret behind every effective bodyweight movement. You'll train it the right way.

4. A Personalized, No-Excuses Training System

No gym? No problem. You'll have a full program you can do at home, at a park, or anywhere with space to move. No expensive gear. No complex routines. Just a clear path you can follow — with enough flexibility to adjust to your schedule and your starting level.

5. Confidence That Comes From Mastery

There's a quiet confidence that grows when you realize, day by day, you're getting stronger on your own terms. You won't need mirrors to validate your progress. You'll feel it — in the way you move, the way you recover, the way you hold yourself. That's the power of calisthenics.

If you read this book cover to cover, follow the progressions, and apply what you learn — even for just a few weeks — you'll begin to shift not only how you train, but how you see your body.

How to Use This Guide

This book is designed to be your complete starting point in calisthenics — not just a list of exercises, but a full framework for how to build strength, mobility, and control from the ground up.

You don't need to read it all at once. But you do need to follow it with intention. Every chapter has a purpose, and each one builds on the last. Here's how to get the most out of it:

Start at the Foundation

If you're a true beginner, do not skip the first two chapters. They walk you through the fundamentals of body mechanics, mindset, and injury prevention. You'll learn how to warm up, how to activate the right muscles, and how to set a foundation that keeps you progressing without setbacks.

Training is more than moving — it's learning how to move well.

Learn the Movements First — Then Train

Each exercise chapter introduces a specific category of training:

- **Mobility & Activation**
- **Core Control**
- **Push Mechanics**
- **Pull Mechanics**
- **Lower Body Strength**
- **Balance & Functional Flow**
- **Cooldown & Flexibility**

Each movement is broken down with clear step-by-step instructions and visual illustrations. Before you jump into a workout routine, take the time to learn these movements. Practice them slowly. Focus on control, not speed.

Use the 30-Day Program as Your Roadmap

In Chapter 10, you'll find a structured 30-day program — laid out week by week with rest days, progression, and built-in variety. This is your blueprint. If you follow it consistently, you'll notice measurable improvement in strength, posture, and body control within just a few weeks.

You can repeat the program multiple times. Each round will feel different because *you* will be different — stronger, more aware, and more capable.

Read, Train, Revisit

This guide is meant to stay with you. Come back to it. Re-read sections as your body changes. The more experienced you become, the more each chapter will teach you. What feels basic today will feel essential tomorrow — that's how good training works.

Calisthenics is simple, but not easy. This book gives you the tools — but it's your commitment that makes the difference. Move with purpose. Read with intention. And trust the structure.

Chapter 1: The Fundamentals of Calisthenics

What Is Calisthenics? Origins, Science, and Benefits

Calisthenics is the art and science of using your own bodyweight to develop strength, control, mobility, and endurance. The movements are simple, but the effects are powerful — and for beginners, it's one of the most efficient and sustainable ways to train.

At its core, calisthenics teaches you how to master the one tool you'll always have: your body.

The Origins: Strength Before Machines

Long before the invention of gyms and resistance machines, people trained with their own bodyweight. Ancient Greek warriors practiced calisthenic drills to prepare for battle. In fact, the word "calisthenics" comes from the Greek words *kallos* (beauty) and *sthenos* (strength) — a system built around graceful, functional power.

Over centuries, bodyweight training has been used by military forces, martial artists, gymnasts, and physical therapists — not just because it works, but because it *lasts*. It doesn't require equipment. It doesn't rely on trends. It's a timeless method of training that adapts to you.

The Science: More Than Just Muscle

Modern research supports what ancient warriors already knew: bodyweight training is effective.

Here's why:

- **Compound Movements:** Most calisthenics exercises recruit multiple muscle groups at once — making them more efficient for building total-body strength and coordination.
- **Neuromuscular Control:** You're not just building muscle — you're training your nervous system to fire the right muscles in the right sequence. That leads to better performance, better posture, and fewer injuries.

- **Joint-Friendly Progression:** Because calisthenics emphasizes movement control over heavy load, it reduces the stress on joints — especially important for beginners and those recovering from injury.

- **Scalable Intensity:** Calisthenics meets you where you are. You can modify movements to fit your level — then progress naturally as your strength improves.

The Benefits: Strength That Goes Beyond the Gym

Calisthenics doesn't just build muscle — it builds capability.

You'll notice improvements in:

- **Strength & Endurance:** From basic squats to extended plank holds, every movement teaches your body to handle its own weight — efficiently and powerfully.

- **Mobility & Flexibility:** Movements like deep squats and hip openers improve your range of motion and unlock stiff joints.

- **Posture & Balance:** As your core and stabilizers strengthen, you'll find yourself standing taller, moving smoother, and feeling more in control.

- **Confidence:** There's something powerful about lifting and controlling your own body. Progress in calisthenics is deeply personal — and the confidence it builds shows up everywhere.

You don't need complicated machines or a wall of dumbbells. You don't need perfect genetics or an athletic background. You need your body, your breath, and a commitment to doing the work — one rep at a time.

That's calisthenics. And by the end of this book, it will be yours.

Understanding Movement Planes and Muscle Chains

If you want to train smarter — not just harder — you need to understand how your body moves. Not just the muscles you see in the mirror, but the patterns and systems that connect everything underneath. That's where movement planes and muscle chains come in.

Don't worry — this isn't about memorizing anatomy. It's about learning how your body works as a unit, so you can train it as one.

The Three Planes of Human Movement

Every movement your body makes happens within one or more of three planes. Think of them like invisible lines that divide how you move through space.

1. **Sagittal Plane (Forward and Backward):**
   This is where most beginners live — squats, lunges, push-ups, and crunches all happen in this plane. It involves forward and backward motion and includes flexion and extension (like bending and straightening your knees or elbows).

2. **Frontal Plane (Side to Side):**
   Movements like side lunges, lateral leg lifts, and jumping jacks happen here. It's crucial for improving balance, stability, and coordination — areas most beginners overlook.

3. **Transverse Plane (Twisting and Rotation):**
   This is the most undertrained plane for most people. Movements like torso twists, rotational planks, and turning lunges train your body to rotate and stabilize — essential for daily life and injury prevention.

A balanced program like this one will include movements from **all three planes**, so you build not just strength, but **functional strength** — the kind that helps you move better in the real world, not just on paper.

Muscle Chains: Why You Should Stop Thinking in Isolation

Most people are taught to think in terms of individual muscles — "train your biceps," "strengthen your abs." But your body doesn't work like that. It moves through **muscle chains** — connected groups of muscles that activate together to create smooth, coordinated motion.

Here are the primary chains you'll engage through calisthenics:

- **Posterior Chain:** The back of your body — hamstrings, glutes, spinal erectors, upper back. This chain drives hip extension, posture, and pulling strength. Think glute bridges, bodyweight rows, dead hangs.

- **Anterior Chain:** The front — quads, abs, chest, shoulders. This chain powers pushing movements and core bracing. Think push-ups, squats, planks.

- **Lateral Chain:** The side-body — obliques, hip abductors, glute medius. This chain stabilizes your pelvis and spine. Think side planks, lateral lunges, bird dogs.

- **Spiral Chain:** This one crosses the body — opposite shoulder to hip — and is essential for rotation, walking, and balance. Think controlled twists, cross-body reach holds, or rotational core work.

Once you stop training muscles in isolation and start training the **systems that move you**, your results multiply. You move better, get stronger faster, and reduce your risk of injury — because you're training your body the way it was designed to move.

Building a Foundation: Balance, Mobility, and Control

Before strength comes control. Before control comes awareness. And before any of that, your body needs the capacity to move freely and stabilize itself under tension. That's why calisthenics starts — and succeeds — with foundation work: balance, mobility, and control.

Skipping these fundamentals is the fastest way to hit a plateau, develop compensations, or worse, get injured. Mastering them? That's how you build strength that actually lasts.

Balance: Your First Layer of Strength

Balance isn't just about standing on one leg — it's your body's ability to remain stable during movement. Every push-up, lunge, or plank you'll do in this book demands balance. And not just from your feet — from your core, hips, shoulders, and nervous system.

Training balance helps you:

- Improve posture and body alignment
- Develop stabilizer muscles most people ignore
- Enhance proprioception — your sense of where your body is in space
- Reduce your risk of falls, stumbles, and joint strain

Without balance, strength becomes unpredictable. You might be able to push, but not land. You might be able to squat, but not recover. That's why we train it early — so every movement that follows is solid.

Mobility: The Prerequisite for Movement

Mobility is often confused with flexibility — but it's not the same. Flexibility is passive. Mobility is active. It's your ability to move a joint through its full range with control.

Think of mobility as the bridge between your joints and your muscles. If your hips are tight, your squat will suffer. If your shoulders are locked up, your push-ups will strain. Mobility isn't optional — it's non-negotiable.

In this book, we incorporate dynamic mobility drills before strength work and recommend focused cool-down sequences to maintain joint health long-term. You'll find your movements becoming easier, smoother, and more natural — often within days of consistent training.

Control: Where Strength Becomes Skill

Muscle without control is just potential. Calisthenics doesn't just build strength — it forces you to own every inch of movement. That's where control comes in.

Control means being able to:

- Start and stop a movement at will
- Maintain alignment throughout the full range
- Recruit the right muscles, at the right time, with the right intensity

When you move with control, you don't just avoid injury — you unlock power. You get stronger, faster. You progress with confidence. And best of all, you build a level of trust in your body that changes how you train forever.

Balance, mobility, and control are not side notes — they are the structure everything else is built on. And in this program, they're not optional add-ons — they're integrated into your workouts from the first chapter to the last.

We don't build strength on dysfunction. We build it on a body that moves well, knows itself, and adapts smartly.

Key Principles: Consistency, Form, and Progression

Results don't come from what you do once in a while. They come from what you repeat — deliberately, consistently, and with attention to detail. Calisthenics rewards those who stay with it. Not for perfection, but for patience. If you want to build a body that performs well, feels strong, and lasts, you'll need to commit to three non-negotiables: **consistency**, **form**, and **progression**.

Consistency: The Real Secret to Progress

The best training plan is the one you can follow. Not just for a week, but for weeks in a row — even when motivation fades. In calisthenics, it's consistency that builds muscle memory, reinforces movement patterns, and teaches your body to adapt.

You don't need to train for hours. You don't need to destroy yourself every session. What you do need is to show up — 3 to 5 times a week — and train with focus. Whether it's a full workout or just a focused core session, the cumulative effect of regular training is where the real change happens.

Discipline beats intensity when you're in this for the long term.

Form: Movement Quality Over Repetition Count

A sloppy rep is a wasted rep — or worse, a path to injury. In calisthenics, proper form is everything. Since you're not relying on external weights, the resistance *is* your body. That means alignment, control, and joint positioning matter more than ever.

This book is built around movement integrity. You'll find step-by-step guidance and visuals for every exercise — not just what to do, but *how* to do it with intention. If your goal is ten push-ups, and you can only do three with perfect form? Do three. That's where the progress lives.

Train clean. Train precisely. Let every rep count.

Progression: Train Smart, Not Just Hard

You won't find random workouts in these pages. You'll find a system. One that adapts as you improve. That's progression — and it's the key to unlocking new strength, safely and sustainably.

Every movement in calisthenics has levels. From incline push-ups to full-range planks, from wall sits to single-leg drills, you'll see how to scale each exercise up or down depending on your current ability.

This is how you avoid plateaus. This is how you prevent burnout. And this is how you stay motivated — not by doing more of the same, but by earning your way to the next challenge.

Together, these three principles — **consistency**, **form**, and **progression** — are what separate short-term effort from long-term transformation. Memorize them. Lean on them. And use them to guide every rep you perform moving forward.

Chapter 2: Readiness & Recovery

Self-Assessment: Where Do You Start?

Before you begin training, you need to understand your body as it is — right now. Not how it used to be, not how you want it to be — but today. This is the most overlooked step in beginner fitness: honest self-assessment. Without it, you either push too hard too soon or hold yourself back when you're more capable than you think.

Here, you won't be judged by numbers on a scale or how fast you can move. This isn't about perfection. It's about understanding your **starting point**, so you can train with precision, not guesswork.

What This Assessment Is (and Isn't)

This is not a fitness test. It's not about proving anything. This is about *gauging movement quality*, *mobility range*, and *basic control*. Calisthenics is about movement mastery — and that begins with knowing what your body can currently handle with proper form.

The goal is to establish a clear baseline across the **four pillars of calisthenics readiness**:

1. **Joint Mobility** — Can you move through essential ranges pain-free?
2. **Core Activation** — Can you engage your core without compensating elsewhere?
3. **Balance & Stability** — Can you hold your body steady without wobbling or overcorrecting?
4. **Basic Strength Control** — Can you move your own body with control and alignment?

Your Readiness Checklist

Perform each of the following **5 simple drills**. There's no equipment needed — just your body, a clear wall or floor space, and honesty.

1. **Deep Bodyweight Squat**
    - Can you lower your hips below your knees while keeping your heels down and chest up?
2. **Straight-Arm Plank Hold (30 seconds)**

- Can you hold a plank with hips level, shoulders over wrists, and without sinking at the lower back?

3. **Wall Shoulder Flexion (Arms Overhead)**
    - Stand with your back flat against a wall. Can you raise both arms overhead to touch the wall without arching your lower back?

4. **Single-Leg Balance (Eyes Open — 20 seconds)**
    - Can you balance on each leg without hopping or using your arms for momentum?

5. **Seated Leg Raise (Core Control)**
    - Sit upright with legs extended. Can you lift one straight leg a few inches off the floor without slouching or leaning back?

Score yourself honestly:

- **Green Light:** Full control and pain-free? You're ready to train.
- **Yellow Light:** Some shakiness or compensation? Start slowly with modifications.
- **Red Light:** Pain or major restriction? Focus on mobility and foundational work first — your strength will catch up.

Why This Matters

Your body keeps score — whether you're paying attention or not. By doing this self-check first, you're giving yourself the chance to train with *precision*, not assumption. You'll also avoid one of the biggest beginner mistakes: trying to copy advanced movements before your body is ready.

Calisthenics rewards those who train what they need — not just what they like.

Take five minutes to run through the checklist. No ego, no rush. Just awareness. Because the more honestly you start, the stronger you finish.

Injury-Proofing the Body

If your body isn't prepared for movement, strength becomes a liability — not an asset. That's why one of the smartest things you can do as a beginner is learn how to **train without breaking down**. In calisthenics, where every rep requires full-body control, injury prevention isn't a bonus — it's built in.

But you have to approach it with intention.

The Most Common Mistakes Beginners Make

Most injuries at the beginner stage come from **rushing past fundamentals** or **repeating poor form**. You don't need heavy weights to get hurt — all it takes is repeated movement under bad alignment or overused joints. Here are the most common patterns that lead to breakdown:

- **Skipping warm-ups:** Jumping into push-ups or planks cold increases risk to your wrists, shoulders, and lower back.
- **Poor shoulder positioning:** In bodyweight training, shoulder instability is one of the top causes of strain — especially during pushing movements.
- **Overloaded joints:** Repeating squats or planks without attention to knee or wrist angles can lead to inflammation over time.
- **Holding your breath:** Breath-holding during effort (known as the Valsalva maneuver) can increase pressure in joints and reduce control.
- **Too much, too soon:** Volume overload — doing too many sets or sessions before your body adapts — often leads to tendon irritation and burnout.

The good news? These are all preventable.

Here's How You Stay Injury-Free While Progressing:

1. Prioritize Joint Prep

Before strength comes mobility. In this book, every workout begins with **joint-friendly warm-ups** that activate muscles and prime your nervous system. Don't skip them — they're not optional.

2. Learn Neutral Alignment

Your spine, neck, and pelvis need to stay in neutral positions during movement. This reduces unnecessary strain and improves control. You'll learn how to "lock in" your form in exercises like planks, squats, and bridges — and carry that awareness into more advanced work later.

3. Strengthen the Small Stabilizers

Your big muscles move you. Your **stabilizers protect you**. That means your rotator cuff, deep core, glutes, and feet — yes, your feet — need to be trained as part of the whole. This book includes movements that challenge balance and joint integrity so you're building from the inside out.

4. Respect Recovery

Injury is often the result of **under-recovery**, not overtraining. You'll find rest days built into the 30-day plan, along with cooldown routines to help your body bounce back stronger. If something feels off — tight, swollen, or painful — listen. Adjust. Rest. Progress is never lost when you're taking care of the system that does the work.

Train for Longevity, Not Just the Next Session

You're not here to train for a week — you're here to build something that lasts. Every rep, every warm-up, every recovery strategy in this book is designed to support that. No shortcuts. No broken bodies. Just smart, progressive, pain-free training.

Protect your body now, and it will reward you with strength you can rely on for life.

Daily Movement Prep: Warm-Up Protocol

Your warm-up isn't just something to "get out of the way." It's your **insurance policy**, your **performance primer**, and your **injury-prevention strategy** — all rolled into one. Done correctly, it prepares your joints, wakes up your nervous system, and sharpens your movement awareness so that every rep that follows is safer and more effective.

In calisthenics, where you're relying entirely on your body's mechanics, **how you move matters just as much as what you do**. And it starts before the workout even begins.

What an Effective Warm-Up Should Do

A warm-up isn't about getting sweaty — it's about preparing your body to move with purpose. In this program, your daily prep is built around four key goals:

1. **Increase circulation** — raise core temperature to promote blood flow to muscles
2. **Activate key stabilizers** — wake up core, glutes, and postural support muscles
3. **Mobilize major joints** — restore usable range in hips, shoulders, spine, and ankles
4. **Reinforce movement patterns** — cue your body to move well before you load it

---

The Structure of This Warm-Up Protocol

Each warm-up takes **5–7 minutes**, requires **zero equipment**, and can be done anywhere. It's short enough to stay consistent, but powerful enough to prepare you for a full-body session.

You'll go through:

- 3 dynamic mobility drills
- 3 muscle activation movements
- 2 core integration drills

This protocol stays the same throughout your beginner phase, and you'll get better at it — faster, cleaner, and more connected. Consider it your movement ritual. Do it before every workout.

What to Expect Next

In the next chapter — **Mobility & Activation Essentials** — you'll find your full warm-up protocol broken down exercise by exercise. Each movement includes:

- A short description of purpose
- Step-by-step instructions
- Professional illustrations showing correct form
- Key coaching points for breathing, alignment, and control

You'll be ready to move, not just through your warm-up, but through your entire workout — with a body that's primed, focused, and safe.

Rest, Recovery, and Overtraining Signals

Training breaks your body down. **Recovery is what builds it back stronger.** If you skip recovery, you stall progress. If you understand it — and use it strategically — you accelerate growth, prevent injury, and stay consistent over the long term.

In calisthenics, where your own body is the weight, fatigue shows up differently than it might in the gym. There's no barbell to drop when you're tired — but there are clear signals your body sends. You just need to know how to read them.

Why Beginners Often Undervalue Recovery

When you're new to training, it's tempting to think more is better. More workouts. More reps. More days in a row. But the truth is, your body doesn't get stronger during your sessions — it gets stronger **after**, when it's resting and rebuilding.

Inconsistent energy, nagging joint soreness, or a plateau in performance are often **not signs that you need to work harder** — they're signs you need to recover better.

Recovery Is Not the Same as Inactivity

Let's be clear: recovery doesn't mean lying on the couch for three days. Smart recovery is active — it includes:

- **Mobility sessions**
- **Light movement (like walking or stretching)**
- **Hydration and proper nutrition**
- **Quality sleep**
- **Breathwork and stress regulation**

These factors reset your nervous system and support muscular repair. That's how you come back stronger — not just rested, but recharged.

How to Recognize Overtraining (Even Without Weights)

Because calisthenics feels "lighter" than lifting weights, it's easy to overlook signs of overuse. Here's what to watch for:

- **Persistent fatigue** that doesn't improve with sleep
- **Decreased performance**, even in basic movements
- **Mood changes** — irritability, anxiety, or low motivation to train
- **Poor sleep** despite feeling exhausted
- **Nagging joint pain** in wrists, shoulders, or knees
- **Resting heart rate increases** over several days

If you're noticing more than one of these, it's a sign your body needs a reset — not a harder workout. Drop back volume, take an extra rest day, or focus on mobility until your system is ready to go again.

How This Program Supports Recovery

You'll notice built-in rest days and varied intensity throughout the 30-day program. These aren't gaps — they're essential pieces of the plan. You'll train 3–5 days per week depending on your level, with each week progressing slightly in complexity, not just volume.

There's also a full **Cooldown & Flexibility chapter** later in the book, designed to speed up recovery and improve how your body feels between sessions.

Train Hard. Recover Smarter.

Beginners who train intelligently always outperform those who train excessively. This book isn't about pushing you to the limit — it's about helping you reach your potential by giving your body what it actually needs to grow.

Respect rest. Prioritize recovery. Listen to the signals.

This is how you stay in the game — and how you win over the long term.

Chapter 3: Mobility & Activation Essentials

Mobility + Activation Exercises

Before you build strength, you need access. Access to your full range of motion. Access to the muscles that stabilize your joints. Access to the breathing patterns that fuel control. That's what this chapter is designed to unlock.

Mobility and activation are your **first layer of training** — the groundwork that every movement in this book is built upon. If you skip this layer, your training becomes compensation: tight hips affecting your squats, weak glutes overloading your knees, or stiff shoulders turning push-ups into pain. That's not strength — that's dysfunction under effort.

But when you start with movement prep, your body responds differently. Everything feels smoother. Your joints move more freely. You begin each session focused, connected, and ready to train — not just sweat.

Why Mobility + Activation Work?

Most beginner injuries and plateaus can be traced back to one of two problems: moving with limited range or moving without control. Mobility gives you the range. Activation gives you the control. Together, they create a body that can move **well**, not just move **more**.

You'll feel the difference almost immediately — hips that open more naturally, a core that engages before your limbs even move, and joints that feel supported instead of strained.

Your first step begins now — not with a heavy rep, but with the small, precise movements that make every rep that follows stronger, safer, and more efficient.

Arm Swings

Purpose

To warm up the shoulders, chest, and upper back while increasing circulation and gently loosening the arms before upper body or full-body sessions.

How to Perform It

1. Stand tall with your feet shoulder-width apart and arms relaxed by your sides.
2. Begin with front-to-back swings: move both arms forward and backward in a smooth, continuous arc, keeping your elbows soft and shoulders relaxed.
3. After 10–15 swings, switch to cross-body swings: open your arms wide, then swing them across your chest, alternating which arm crosses over the top.
4. Maintain a steady rhythm and stay upright throughout the movement.
5. Perform each variation for 20–30 seconds, or until your shoulders feel mobile and warm.

Execution Keys

- Keep your **core gently braced** to avoid arching your lower back.
- Let your **shoulders and arms move naturally** — don't force range or overreach.
- Breathe comfortably and rhythmically.
- Focus on **fluid motion**, not speed.

⚠ **Safety Tip**

Avoid swinging too aggressively — use a relaxed, controlled range to prevent shoulder strain.

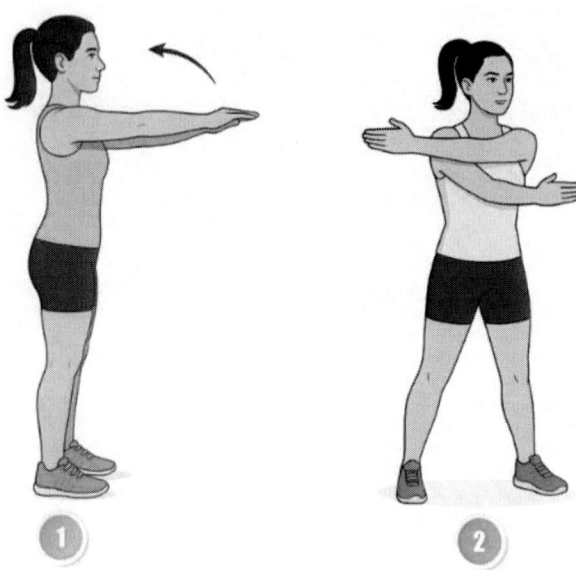

Why It Matters

Arm swings activate the muscles around your shoulder girdle, stimulate circulation, and help reset posture before demanding upper body work. This simple drill promotes joint lubrication, improves mobility, and mentally primes you to train — all without causing fatigue. It's one of the most effective low-intensity warm-up tools for beginners and experienced movers alike.

Standing Hip Openers

Purpose

To mobilize the hips, loosen tight hip flexors, and prepare the lower body for squatting, lunging, or stepping movements.

How to Perform It

1. Stand tall with feet hip-width apart and hands lightly resting on your hips or holding a wall or chair for balance.
2. Shift your weight onto your left leg and lift your right knee up to hip level in front of you.
3. Slowly rotate your right knee outward in a wide arc, as if opening a gate — keeping your torso upright.
4. Reverse the motion to bring the leg back to center and lower it down with control.
5. Repeat 6–8 reps on one side before switching to the opposite leg.

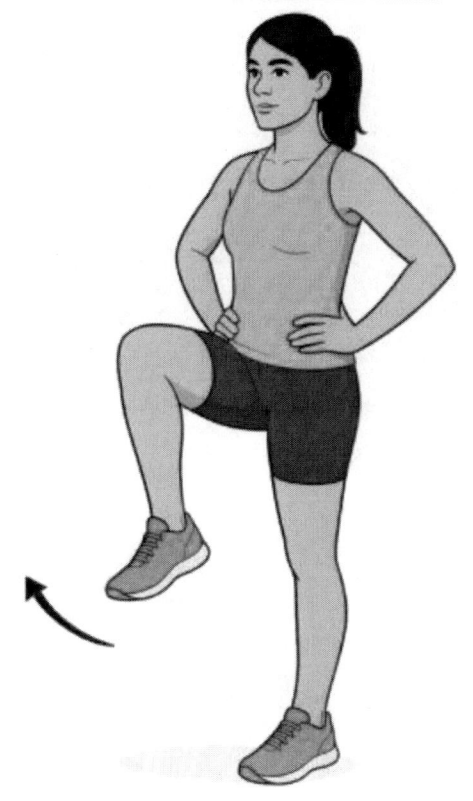

Execution Keys

- Keep your **core engaged** to prevent leaning or twisting.
- Move your leg like a controlled pendulum — not a swing.
- Make the circle **wide but smooth**, staying within your comfortable range.
- Maintain a **tall spine** throughout; don't hunch forward.
- Use a chair or wall if your balance wavers — stability over strain.

⚠ Safety Tip

If you feel pinching in the hip or lower back, reduce the range of motion and move more slowly — don't force the arc.

Why It Matters

Tight hips limit how well you can squat, lunge, or even walk efficiently. This movement gently opens up the hip joint, improves circulation, and helps restore your natural range of motion.

Leg Swings

Purpose

To increase dynamic flexibility in the hips and hamstrings while improving hip joint lubrication and activating the lower body before strength movements.

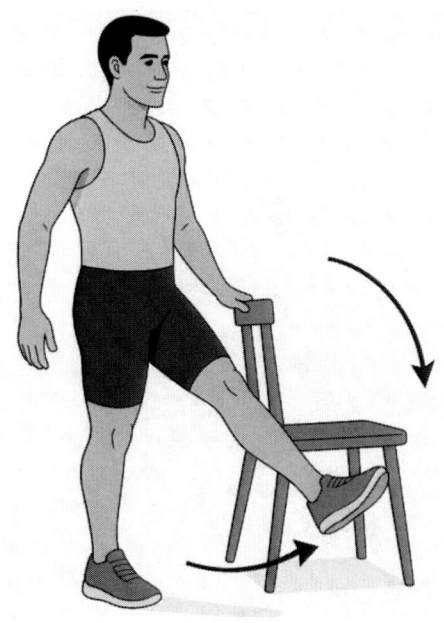

How to Perform It

1. Stand beside a wall, sturdy chair, or rail for support, feet shoulder-width apart.//
2. Shift your weight onto your left foot and lift your right leg slightly off the floor.
3. Begin swinging your right leg **forward and backward** in a controlled arc — keeping it straight but not locked at the knee.
4. Focus on keeping your upper body tall and relaxed, using the wall or support to maintain balance.
5. Perform 10–15 swings, then switch legs.

Execution Keys

- Let the movement come from the **hip joint**, not the lower back.
- Keep your **torso upright** — avoid leaning forward or back.
- Breathe rhythmically and swing with **control**, not speed.
- Engage your **core gently** to stay stable throughout the movement.
- Allow your leg to move freely, but stop short of any jerking or snapping.

⚠ Safety Tip

Avoid overextending your leg behind you — this can strain your lower back. Keep the swing natural and within your current flexibility range.

Why It Matters

Leg swings are a dynamic way to prepare the hips and hamstrings for work. They help restore range of motion, improve joint circulation, and activate the stabilizers needed for lunges, squats, and jumps. By swinging in a controlled arc, you're training your nervous system to move dynamically while maintaining balance and posture — key components of effective calisthenics.

Wrist Rolls & Finger Pulses

Purpose

To warm up and mobilize the wrists, fingers, and forearms — reducing tension and preparing the upper extremities for weight-bearing and grip-based movements.

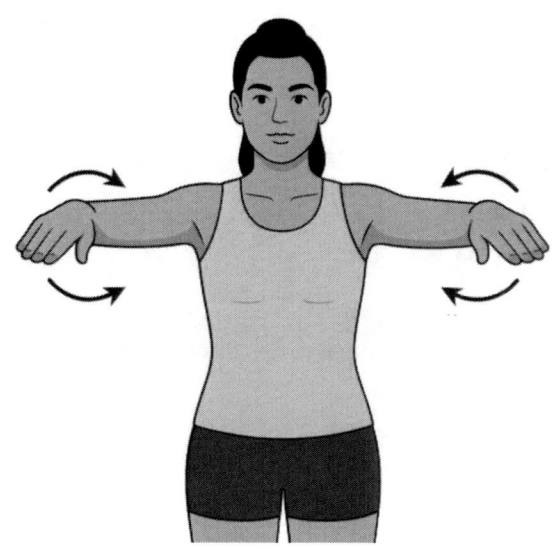

How to Perform It

1. Stand or sit tall with your arms extended in front of you at shoulder height, elbows soft and hands relaxed.

2. Begin rotating both wrists slowly in small circles — **5–8 rotations clockwise**, then **5–8 counterclockwise**.

3. After the rolls, spread your fingers wide, then gently **pulse them closed** into a soft fist and open again.

4. Repeat the **open-close pulses** 10–15 times with control, keeping the shoulders relaxed.

5. Shake out your hands gently afterward to release any tension.

Execution Keys

- Focus on **slow, full wrist circles** — avoid rushing the motion.
- Keep your **fingers long and active** during the open/close pulses.
- Relax your **neck and shoulders** — don't let tension creep upward.
- If seated, maintain upright posture with feet flat on the floor.
- Synchronize your breath with the movement to stay focused and calm.

⚠ Safety Tip

If you feel a snapping or grinding sensation in your wrists, reduce the range of your circles and move slower. Never force rotation.

Why It Matters

Wrist mobility and finger control are critical in calisthenics — especially in movements like planks, push-ups, and downward-loaded positions. Most beginners neglect this area until discomfort shows up. This simple prep drill keeps your wrists supple, your grip strong, and your hand joints moving well. Think of it as insurance for every push, press, or hold that follows.

Cat-Cow Flow

Purpose

To mobilize the spine, relieve tension in the back and neck, and improve body awareness through rhythmic spinal flexion and extension.

How to Perform It

1. Begin on all fours in a tabletop position: hands directly under shoulders, knees under hips, spine in a neutral position.

2. Inhale as you gently drop your belly toward the floor, lifting your tailbone and chest — gaze slightly forward. This is **Cow**.

3. Exhale as you round your spine upward, tucking your pelvis and drawing your chin toward your chest. This is **Cat**.

4. Continue alternating between Cow and Cat with each breath — move slowly and smoothly.

5. Complete 6–10 full cycles, maintaining control and flow throughout.

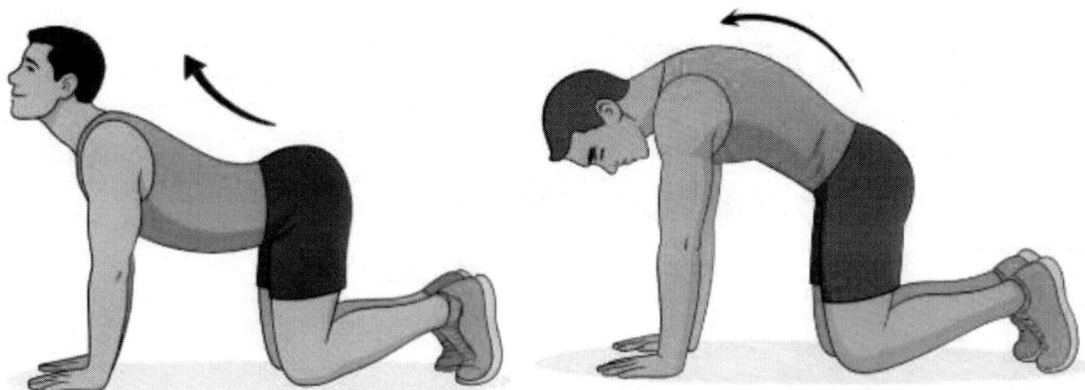

Execution Keys

- Keep your **hands and knees grounded** — avoid shifting weight forward or backward.
- Lead the motion from the **pelvis**, then allow the rest of the spine to follow.

⚠ **Safety Tip**

Avoid forcing extreme arching or rounding. Move gently and stay within a comfortable range — especially if you have any spinal sensitivity.

Deep Squat

Purpose

To open the hips, ankles, and lower back while improving joint flexibility and postural control in the bottom squat position.

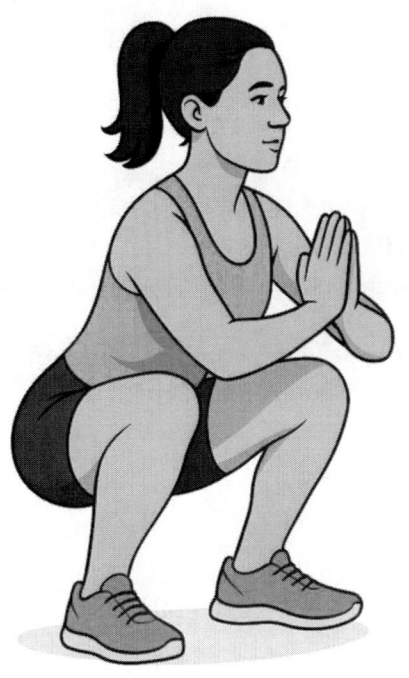

How to Perform It

1. Stand with your feet slightly wider than hip-width apart, toes turned out gently (15–30 degrees).

2. Slowly lower into a deep squat by bending your knees and hips, keeping your heels grounded throughout.

3. Let your hips sink below your knees if possible, maintaining an upright chest and relaxed arms.

4. If needed, place your hands on the floor in front of you or bring your palms together at your chest (prayer position).

5. Hold for 20–30 seconds, breathing deeply. Shift your weight slightly side to side to gently open your hips further.

Execution Keys

- Keep your **heels flat** — avoid lifting them off the ground.
- Engage your **core lightly** to support your lower back.
- Keep your **chest lifted** and avoid collapsing forward.
- Use **elbows to gently press knees outward** if in prayer position.

⚠ Safety Tip

Don't force depth. If your knees or lower back feel strained, reduce the squat depth or use a wall or chair for support.

Why It Matters

The deep squat is a foundational mobility position that improves flexibility in the hips, ankles, and lower spine. It restores a natural range of motion that's essential for squatting, lunging, and maintaining joint health long-term. Holding this position daily helps counteract tightness from prolonged sitting and builds strength in the body's most primal movement pattern.

Spinal Rolls

Purpose

To mobilize the spine segment by segment, improve postural awareness, and gently release tension in the back, neck, and hamstrings.

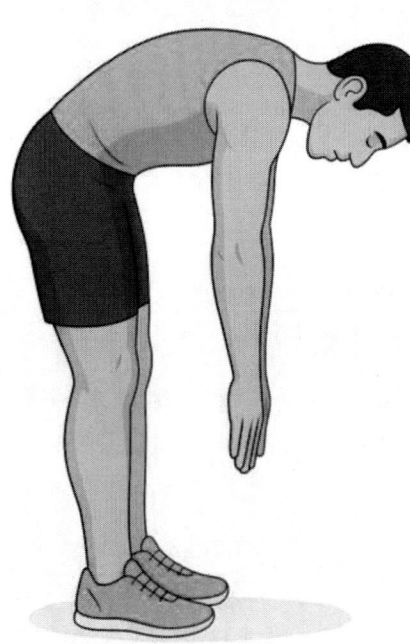

How to Perform It

1. Stand tall with your feet hip-width apart, arms relaxed by your sides, and knees slightly soft.

2. Inhale to prepare. As you exhale, slowly begin to **roll down through your spine**, starting with your head, then neck, shoulders, and upper back — one vertebra at a time.

3. Let your arms hang naturally as you continue folding forward, stopping where your flexibility allows (knees may bend slightly).

4. Pause briefly at the bottom. On an inhale, slowly **reverse the motion**, stacking the spine back up from the lower back to the head.

5. Repeat 4–6 times, keeping the motion smooth and controlled throughout.

Execution Keys

- Lead with the **head and neck**, not the arms — this is a spinal movement, not a hamstring stretch.
- Keep your **core lightly engaged** to support your lower back on the way up.
- Breathe slowly and rhythmically: exhale during the roll down, inhale as you rise.
- Let gravity guide the descent — don't pull or bounce.

⚠ Safety Tip

If you feel dizziness or pulling in the lower back, reduce the range and move slower. Keep your eyes closed only if balance is steady.

Why It Matters

Spinal rolls restore mobility between vertebrae and reconnect you to the rhythm of your body. They reduce stiffness in the back, decompress the spine, and ease tension from long hours of sitting or poor posture. For calisthenics, they also reawaken postural muscles that support planks, push-ups, and controlled standing movements.

Hamstring Scoops

Purpose

To dynamically stretch the hamstrings while improving hip hinge awareness and activating the posterior chain through controlled, sweeping motion.

How to Perform It

1. Stand tall with your feet hip-width apart and arms relaxed by your sides.
2. Step your right foot forward, heel on the ground, toes pointing up.
3. With a **flat back**, hinge at your hips and reach both hands down toward your forward foot, "scooping" along the floor in one smooth motion.
4. Rise back to standing and return your foot to starting position.
5. Alternate legs, performing 6–10 scoops per side in a steady, flowing rhythm.

Execution Keys

- Keep your **spine long and flat** — avoid rounding your back.
- Hinge from the **hips**, not the waist, to feel the stretch in your hamstrings.
- Reach with both hands together in a smooth, downward arc — imagine scooping air.
- Keep your front leg **straight but not locked**, and avoid bouncing.
- Move with a steady tempo, coordinating movement with breath.

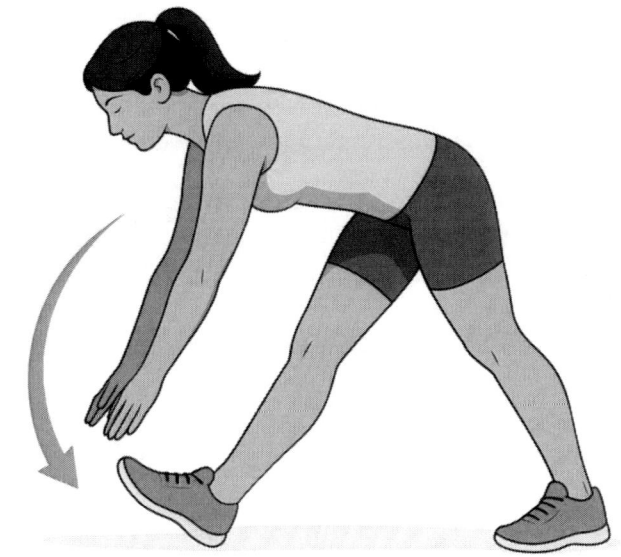

⚠ Safety Tip

Avoid snapping or jerking into the stretch — move only within your comfortable range to prevent hamstring strain.

Why It Matters

Dynamic hamstring scoops activate and lengthen the back of the legs, improve hip mobility, and reinforce proper hinge mechanics — all critical for squats, lunges, and forward-bending movements. They also serve as a low-impact primer for lower-body training, helping you unlock tightness without risking static overstretching before movement.

Chapter 4: Core Foundation & Stability

Core-Specific Exercises

Your core isn't just your abs — it's the center of everything you do. In calisthenics, your ability to move with control, balance, and precision depends heavily on how well your core functions. A weak core shows up everywhere: in unstable planks, poor posture, low back pain, and loss of power during full-body movements.

This chapter is about more than aesthetics. It's about building **real core function** — from the deep stabilizers around your spine to the obliques, glutes, and hip flexors that anchor your movement. You'll learn how to brace, breathe, and engage correctly — without compensation or strain.

What You'll Train in This Chapter

This section includes **core-focused exercises**, all designed to:

- Activate your deep core muscles
- Improve spinal stability
- Build control during dynamic and static movements
- Support full-body calisthenics progressions (push-ups, planks, hollow holds)

Each exercise includes:

- A clear purpose
- Step-by-step instructions
- Execution Keys and Safety Tips

These are not just "ab workouts." They're movement primers, postural correctives, and control builders. The work you do here will directly impact every chapter that follows.

Dead Bug

Purpose

To activate deep core stabilizers, improve coordination, and teach controlled limb movement while keeping the spine neutral — a foundational drill for all calisthenics work.

How to Perform It

1. Lie flat on your back with your knees bent at 90 degrees above your hips and arms extended straight toward the ceiling.
2. Engage your core and flatten your lower back into the floor.
3. Slowly extend your **left leg forward** and **right arm overhead**, keeping both just above the floor.
4. Pause briefly, then return to the starting position with control.
5. Repeat on the opposite side, alternating sides for 8–10 reps per side.

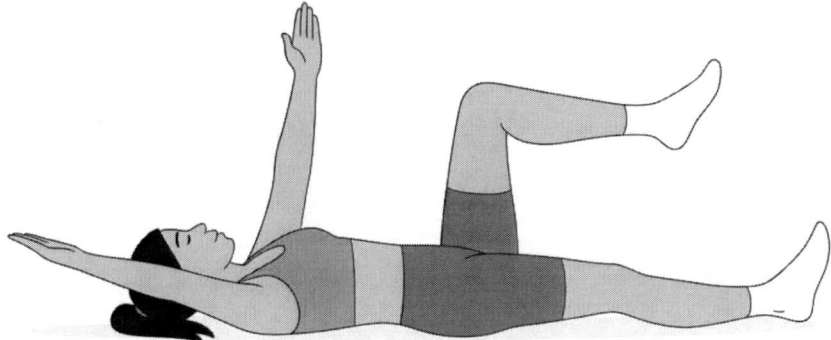

Execution Keys

- Press your **lower back into the floor** throughout the movement — no arching.
- Move **slowly and with control** — the goal is precision, not speed.
- Extend only as far as you can without losing spinal contact.

⚠ Safety Tip

If your back lifts off the floor during the extension, shorten the range of motion and refocus on core engagement — never force full extension if it compromises form.

Why It Matters

This movement trains your body to stabilize your spine while the arms and legs move independently — a core skill in nearly every bodyweight exercise. It builds deep, functional strength that protects your back, improves coordination, and lays the groundwork for advanced calisthenics patterns like hollow holds and planks. When performed correctly, it's one of the most effective beginner core drills available.

Hollow Body Hold

Purpose

To develop deep core tension, spinal stability, and total-body control — essential for progressing into advanced calisthenics movements like leg raises, planks, and levers.

How to Perform It

1. Lie flat on your back with your legs extended and arms reaching overhead.//
2. Press your lower back firmly into the floor and engage your core.
3. Lift your **shoulder blades** off the floor and raise your **legs** 6–12 inches off the ground, keeping them straight and together.
4. At the same time, lift your arms off the floor and hold them extended overhead, biceps near your ears.
5. Maintain this position for 10–20 seconds to start, increasing duration as your control improves.

Execution Keys

- Focus on **maintaining spinal contact** — your lower back should stay glued to the floor.
- Keep your **head in line with your spine**, eyes looking up.
- Engage your thighs and glutes to support leg position.
- Breathe in short, controlled breaths — avoid holding your breath.
- Start with arms at your sides if overhead is too difficult initially.

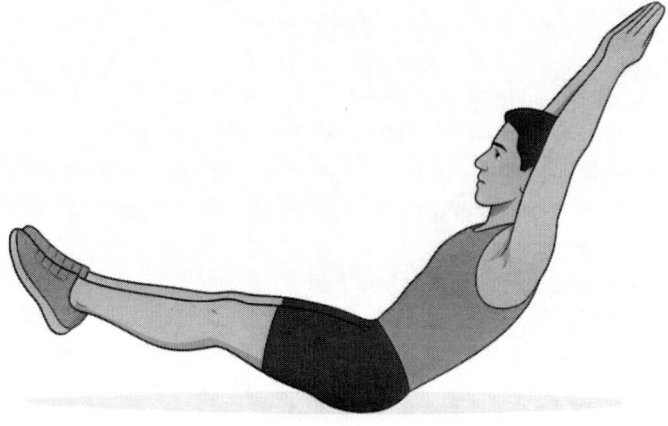

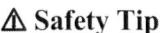 **Safety Tip**

If your lower back arches off the floor, lower your arms and legs slightly or bend your knees to reduce the lever length and stay in control.

Why It Matters

The hollow body hold teaches full-body tension — the kind you need in push-ups, planks, and nearly every calisthenics skill. It's not just an ab exercise — it's a position that rewires your nervous system to engage your core reflexively. Mastering this hold unlocks cleaner form, better control, and faster progression across the entire program.

Bird Dog Reach

Purpose

To build core stability, balance, and spinal alignment through cross-body control — activating deep stabilizers in the abs, glutes, and back.

How to Perform It

1. Start in a tabletop position on all fours, with your hands under shoulders and knees under hips.
2. Engage your core and maintain a neutral spine.
3. Slowly extend your **right arm forward** and **left leg straight back**, keeping both parallel to the floor.
4. Pause for 2–3 seconds while maintaining balance and full-body tension.
5. Return to the starting position and repeat on the other side.
6. Perform 6–8 reps per side, alternating slowly and with full control.

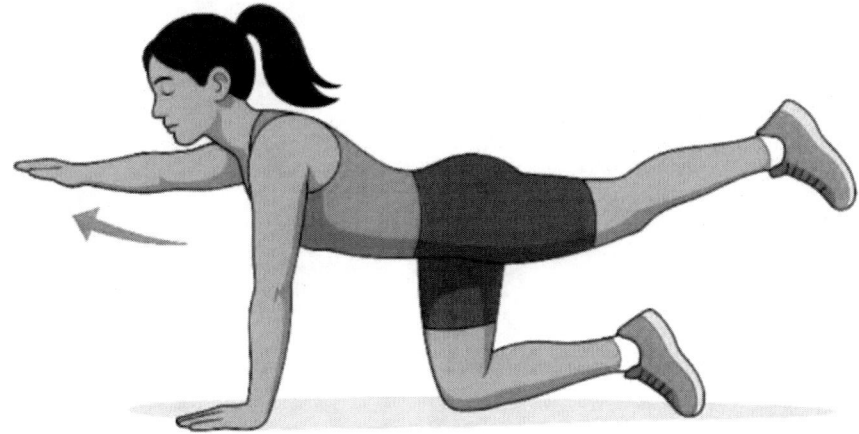

Execution Keys

- Keep your **hips square** — avoid letting one side rotate or dip.
- Maintain a **long line** from fingertips to toes when extended.
- Keep your **gaze down** — don't lift your head.
- Exhale as you extend, inhale as you return.
- Move with slow, intentional rhythm — rushing defeats the purpose.

⚠ Safety Tip

If your lower back arches or your hips wobble, reduce your range of motion or perform just the arm or leg extension until control improves.

Seated Knee Lift Hold

Purpose

To activate the lower abdominals, improve core-limb coordination, and reinforce posture and hip flexor control in a low-impact seated position.

How to Perform It

1. Sit tall on the floor with your legs extended in front of you and your arms resting at your sides for support.

2. Place your fingertips lightly on the floor beside your hips, keeping your spine long and chest lifted.

3. Inhale to prepare. On your exhale, **lift one knee** a few inches off the floor, keeping your foot hovering above the ground.

4. Hold the lifted position for **3–5 seconds**, keeping your core engaged and posture upright.

5. Lower the leg slowly and repeat on the other side.

6. Alternate legs for 6–8 reps per side.

Execution Keys

- Avoid leaning back — keep your **torso upright** and tall.

- Use minimal hand pressure — the lift should come from **core and hip flexor activation**, not arm support.

- Keep your **foot off the ground** during the hold, even if only slightly.

- Breathe slowly and maintain tension throughout the movement.

- If needed, bend your supporting knee slightly for added balance.

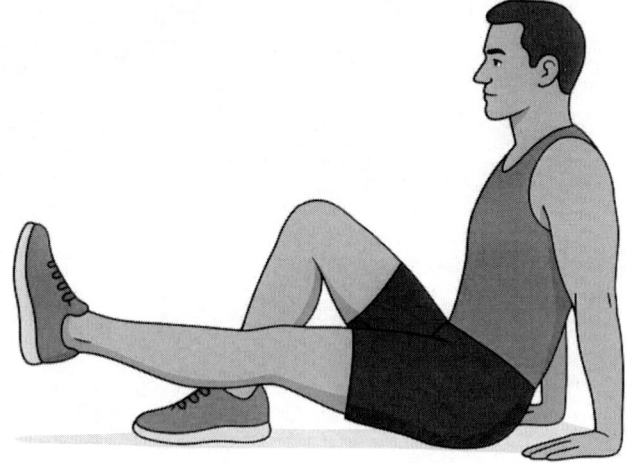

⚠ **Safety Tip**

If you feel strain in your lower back, reduce the height of your lift or place a small rolled towel under your hips for elevation.

Mountain Taps

Purpose

To activate the deep core while developing shoulder stability, total-body coordination, and dynamic control from a high plank position.

How to Perform It

1. Begin in a strong high plank position: hands under shoulders, feet hip-width apart, and body in a straight line from head to heels.

2. Engage your core and glutes to maintain a stable plank.

3. Slowly lift your **right foot** a few inches off the floor and tap it gently forward toward your right hand.

4. Return the foot to plank position and repeat on the left side.

5. Continue alternating legs for **10–12 slow, deliberate reps per side**, keeping your upper body stable throughout.

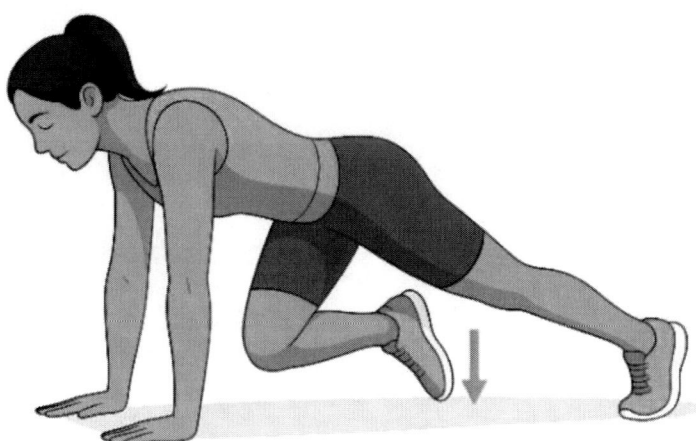

Execution Keys

- Keep your **hips low and square** — avoid bouncing or twisting.
- Move **one leg at a time** — full control is more important than speed.
- Maintain pressure through your palms to stabilize your shoulders.

⚠ Safety Tip

If your hips sag or shoulders fatigue quickly, pause and reset between reps or shorten your tap range to maintain good form.

Lying Windshield Wipers

Purpose

To develop rotational core strength, improve spinal control, and increase mobility through the obliques, hips, and lower back.

How to Perform It

1. Lie on your back with your arms extended out to the sides in a **"T"** position for stability.

2. Raise both legs together toward the ceiling, keeping them straight or slightly bent.

3. Engage your core and slowly lower your **legs to the right side**, stopping just before they touch the floor.

4. Pause briefly, then use your core to pull your legs back to center.

5. Repeat to the left side. Perform **6–8 reps per side**, keeping the motion smooth and even.

Execution Keys

- Keep your **shoulders flat** on the ground throughout — do not twist your upper body.

- Control the descent with your **core**, not momentum.

- The range of motion should allow control — don't drop legs all the way to the ground unless you're advanced.

- Move both legs as a **unit** — avoid letting one side lag behind.

- Exhale during the twist, inhale as you return to center.

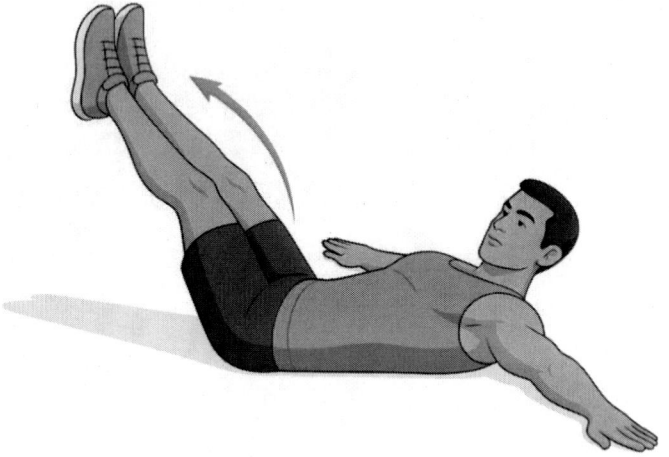

⚠ Safety Tip

Avoid this movement if you have existing lower back pain. If needed, bend your knees to reduce leverage and protect your spine.

Why It Matters

Lying windshield wipers challenge your body's ability to resist and control rotation — a key function of the obliques and deep core muscles. It's especially useful for improving spinal integrity, dynamic stability, and functional strength in twisting movements. For calisthenics beginners, it builds rotational awareness and mobility while reinforcing proper bracing under motion.

Seated Leg Extensions

Purpose

To strengthen the hip flexors and quadriceps while reinforcing core control and postural awareness in a low-impact seated position.

How to Perform It

1. Sit upright on the floor with your legs extended and hands resting lightly beside your hips for balance.
2. Engage your core and lift your **right leg** a few inches off the floor, keeping it fully extended.
3. Without letting your heel drop, **lift and lower** the leg up and down in small, controlled pulses (3–5 inches in range).
4. Perform 8–10 reps, then switch to the left leg.
5. Keep your chest tall and spine neutral throughout the movement.

Execution Keys

- Sit on a **firm surface** to maintain posture and range.
- Keep your **leg fully extended** — avoid bending the knee.
- Engage your **lower abdominals** to support spinal stability.
- Control each lift — **no bouncing or swinging**.
- Exhale during the lift, inhale as you lower.

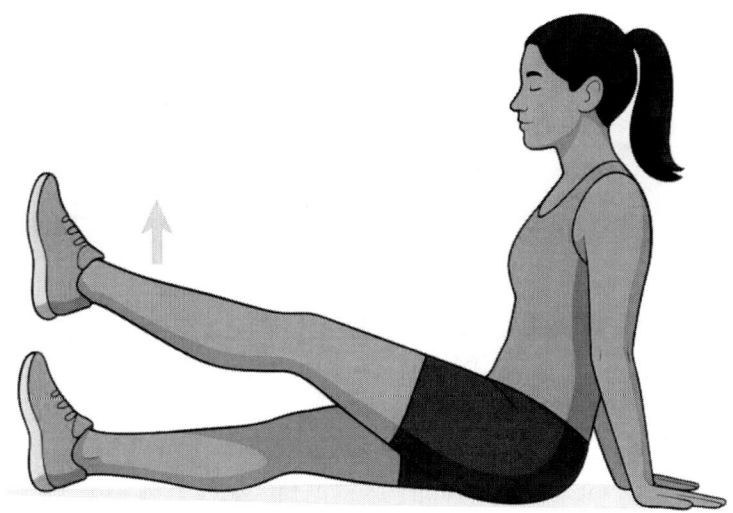

⚠ Safety Tip

If you feel tension in the lower back or hip joint, reduce your leg height or place your hands slightly behind you for more support.

Why It Matters

Seated leg extensions improve control in the hip flexors and quads — critical for mastering straight-leg movements like L-sits, hanging leg raises, and toe touches. They also challenge your core's ability to stabilize your spine in a tall seated position. As a foundational isometric-plus-dynamic drill, it builds control and strength without the need for any equipment.

Plank Push-Up

Purpose

To develop upper body and core strength, shoulder stability, and seamless coordination by transitioning between two foundational bodyweight positions.

How to Perform It

1. Start in a strong **elbow plank** position with your forearms on the floor, elbows under shoulders, and feet hip-width apart.

2. Engage your core and glutes to keep your body in a straight line from head to heels.

3. Shift your weight slightly forward and **place your right hand on the floor**, followed by your left, pushing up into a **high push-up plank**.

4. Pause briefly, maintaining full-body tension.

5. Reverse the motion by lowering back down to your right forearm, then your left, returning to the elbow plank.

6. Alternate the leading arm each rep. Perform 6–10 slow, controlled reps.

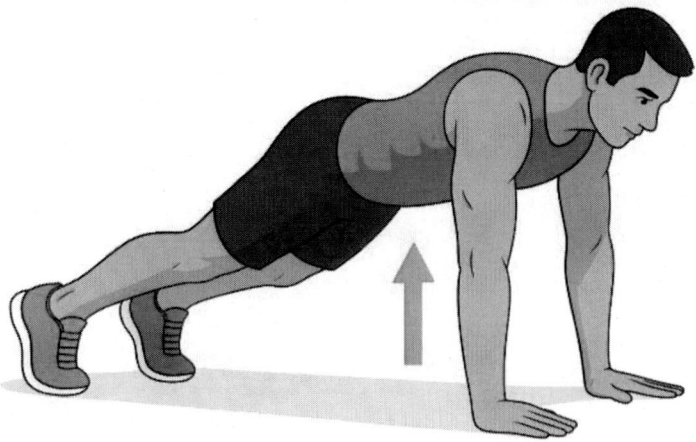

Execution Keys

- Keep your **hips square** — avoid twisting or tilting side to side.

- Move **with control**, not speed — especially during the lowering phase.

- Maintain a **straight spine** and firm shoulder alignment.

- Breathe steadily, exhaling as you press up, inhaling as you lower.

⚠ **Safety Tip**

If you feel strain in your lower back or wrists, drop to your knees while maintaining plank alignment, or reduce reps until strength improves.

Why It Matters

This transition builds dynamic shoulder and core strength while reinforcing control under load. It mimics real-life pushing demands and prepares the body for more advanced calisthenics transitions like planche progressions or elevated planks. When performed slowly and with precision, it's one of the most effective total-body drills for strength and control — no equipment required.

Supine Leg Slide

Purpose

To activate the deep core and hip flexors while reinforcing proper pelvic control and neutral spine alignment — ideal for beginners building foundational strength.

How to Perform It

1. Lie flat on your back with your knees bent, feet flat on the floor, and arms resting beside your body.
2. Engage your core and press your lower back gently into the floor.
3. Slowly **extend your right leg** along the floor, sliding the heel forward until the leg is fully straight.
4. Pause briefly, then slide the leg back to the starting position.
5. Repeat with the **left leg**, alternating for 8–10 reps per side.

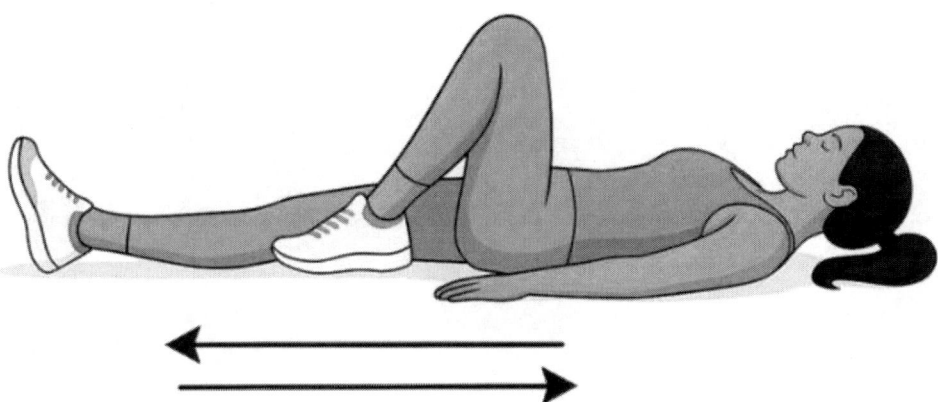

Execution Keys

- Maintain **constant core tension** to prevent your back from arching.
- Keep your **heel in contact with the floor** throughout the slide.
- Move slowly and **without jerking** — the slower, the better.
- Inhale as you slide the leg out, exhale as you return.

⚠ Safety Tip

If your lower back lifts off the floor during the slide, reduce the range of motion or bend the extended leg slightly to stay in control.

Reverse Tabletop Hold

Purpose

To strengthen the posterior chain — especially glutes, hamstrings, shoulders, and spinal extensors — while improving posture and shoulder mobility through active lifting.

How to Perform It

1. Sit on the floor with your **knees bent**, feet flat and hip-width apart, and hands placed slightly behind your hips, fingers pointing toward your feet.

2. Press through your hands and heels to **lift your hips** upward until your body forms a tabletop: shoulders, hips, and knees in a straight line.

3. Keep your head in a neutral position or gently drop it back if comfortable.

4. Squeeze your glutes and hold the top position for **15–30 seconds**.

5. Lower with control and repeat for 2–3 rounds.

Execution Keys

- Spread weight evenly between **hands and feet** — don't overload wrists.

- Engage your **glutes and hamstrings** to elevate hips, not your lower back.

- Keep your **chest open** and shoulder blades gently drawn together.

- Maintain a straight line from knees to shoulders at the top.

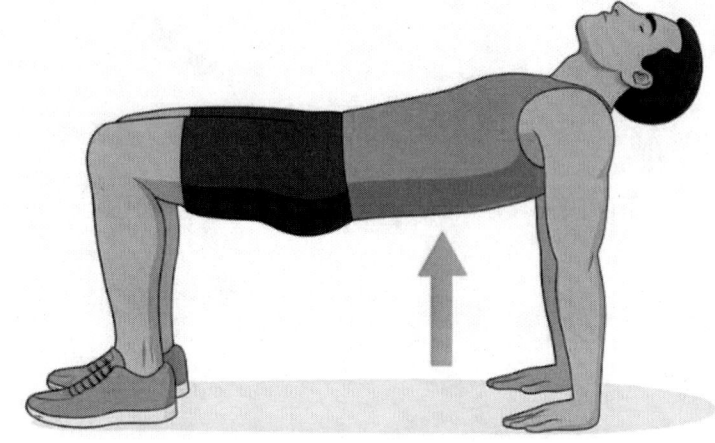

⚠ Safety Tip

Avoid letting your shoulders collapse or overextending your neck. If you experience wrist discomfort, slightly turn your hands outward or elevate your palms on yoga blocks.

Why It Matters

This is more than a stretch — it's a full-body isometric that trains active shoulder extension, glute activation, and spinal opening. For calisthenics beginners, the reverse tabletop hold counters hours of slouching and screens by building postural strength and mobility at the same time. It lays the groundwork for dips, backbends, and explosive posterior chain power.

Chapter 5: Push Mechanics for Beginners

Push-Based Movements

There's a unique confidence that comes from being able to push your own body away from the floor — and calisthenics is built on that foundation. Whether it's a push-up, a wall-assisted dip, or a basic arm extension, pushing strength is essential not just for aesthetics, but for structural control, joint protection, and functional ability.

But here's the reality: many beginners approach push-based training the wrong way — either rushing through poor form, overloading before they're ready, or copying advanced routines without understanding mechanics. This chapter rewires that approach.

We'll begin by focusing on the building blocks of **push mechanics** — how your shoulders, chest, triceps, and core work together to press your body with integrity. These are not just exercises; they're carefully sequenced movements that teach you to generate power while maintaining full-body tension and joint alignment.

What You'll Learn and Train in This Chapter

- Master the **alignment and technique** behind safe, strong pushing patterns
- Build control through **isometric holds, regressions, and floor-based drills**
- Improve **scapular mobility and shoulder stability**
- Learn how to prepare for full push-ups and bodyweight dips — safely
- Rewire posture by integrating strength with position

This isn't about pumping out reps. It's about owning your movement from the ground up — pushing with precision, posture, and purpose. Whether you've never done a push-up in your life or you're rebuilding after injury, this chapter gives you everything you need to start pushing forward with control and confidence.

Wall Push-Ups

Purpose

To build foundational upper body strength, improve scapular control, and reinforce proper push-up alignment in a low-resistance, beginner-friendly format.

How to Perform It

1. Stand facing a sturdy wall at about arm's length, with your feet hip-width apart.
2. Place your palms flat on the wall at shoulder height and slightly wider than shoulder-width, fingers pointing upward.
3. Engage your core and glutes to maintain a straight posture from head to heels.
4. Slowly **bend your elbows** to lower your chest toward the wall, keeping your elbows at a 45° angle from your sides.
5. Pause just before your nose reaches the wall, then **press back** to the starting position.
6. Perform 10–15 slow, controlled repetitions.

Execution Keys

- Keep your **body in one straight line** — don't let your hips sag or back arch.
- Actively press through your palms and **feel your shoulder blades glide** along your back.
- Don't rush — a **3-second down, 1-second up** rhythm builds control.
- Exhale as you push away from the wall, inhale as you lower.

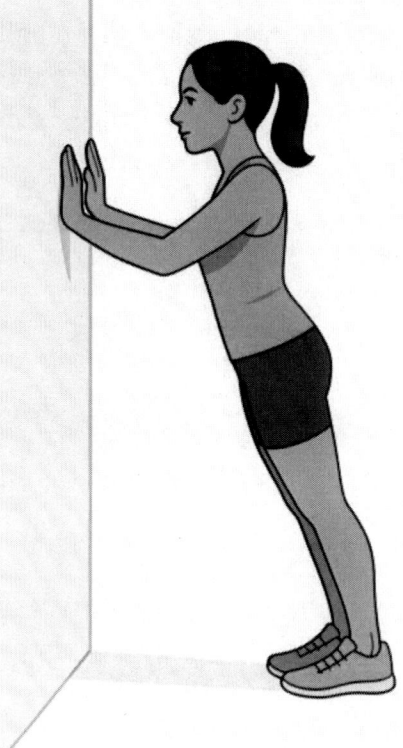

⚠ Safety Tip

If you feel wrist discomfort, lower your hand placement slightly or shift to fists against the wall to reduce pressure.

Why It Matters

Wall push-ups are the safest, most scalable way to begin developing pushing strength, especially for those with limited upper body experience or recovering from injury. They teach you how to brace your core, align your joints, and engage the chest, shoulders, and triceps without the risk of floor-based strain. Mastering this version is the key to progressing confidently into incline and full push-ups.

Incline Push-Ups

Purpose

To strengthen the chest, shoulders, triceps, and core while safely progressing from wall push-ups toward standard floor push-ups.

How to Perform It

1. Stand facing a sturdy surface like a countertop, bench, or heavy chair.
2. Place your hands on the edge, slightly wider than shoulder-width, and walk your feet back until your body forms a straight line from head to heels.
3. Brace your core and glutes. Keep your elbows at a 45° angle to your body.
4. Lower your chest toward the edge by bending your elbows, maintaining full-body tension.
5. Stop just before your chest touches the surface, then press back up to full arm extension.
6. Perform **8–12 controlled reps**, adjusting foot position to manage difficulty.

Execution Keys

- Choose a surface that doesn't move — **stability is non-negotiable**.
- Keep your **hips level** and avoid sagging or arching the lower back.
- Elbows should not flare out — maintain the natural push-up angle.
- Inhale on the descent, exhale as you push up.
- Slower is stronger — **focus on tension, not speed**.

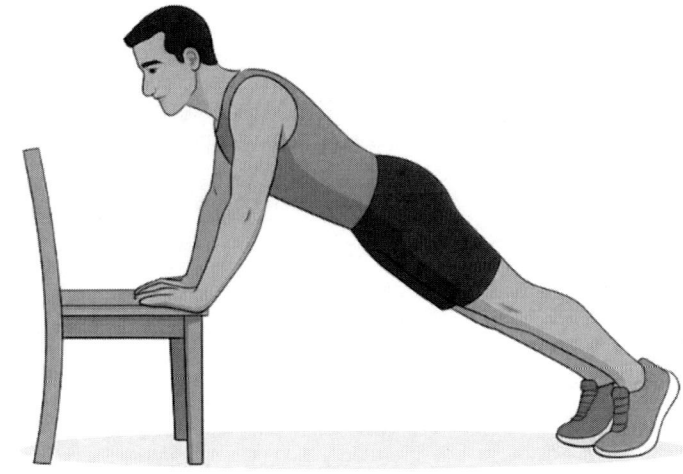

⚠ Safety Tip

Avoid using lightweight or unstable furniture. If you feel shoulder discomfort, slightly narrow your hand position and reduce depth.

Why It Matters

Incline push-ups provide the perfect stepping stone from wall variations to full ground-based push-ups. By adjusting the incline height, you control resistance while training full-body form and upper body strength under load. This movement builds the exact mechanics needed for traditional push-ups — without the discouragement or joint strain of starting from the floor too soon.

Kneeling Push-Ups

Purpose

To build pressing strength and upper body coordination while reducing the load on the core and lower body — an ideal transition from wall or incline push-ups to standard floor variations.

How to Perform It

1. Begin on all fours, then shift your hands forward until your body forms a diagonal line from shoulders to knees.

2. Place your hands slightly wider than shoulder-width, fingers spread, and **draw your shoulder blades slightly together**.

3. Engage your **core and glutes** to stabilize your spine.

4. Lower your chest toward the floor by bending your elbows at a 45° angle.

5. Pause just above the floor, then push back up to full extension.

6. Perform **8–12 reps**, maintaining alignment throughout.

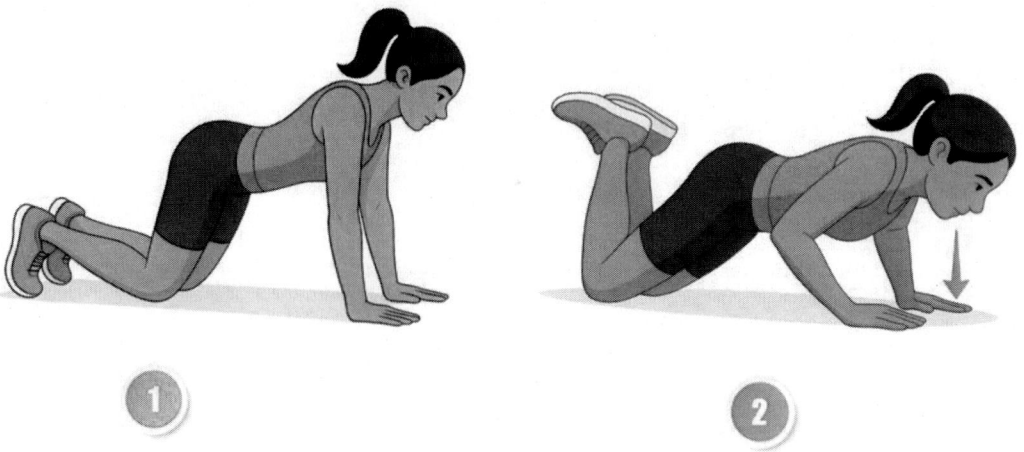

Execution Keys

- Don't just "drop" into the movement — control both the **lowering and pressing phases**.
- Keep your **hips from collapsing** — your torso should move as one piece.
- Adjust your hand placement if you feel wrist pressure.
- Exhale as you press up; inhale as you lower.

⚠ Safety Tip

If your wrists are sensitive, place a folded towel or yoga mat under them, or rotate your hands slightly outward to reduce strain.

Negative Push-Ups

Purpose

To build strength, control, and endurance in the push-up pattern by focusing on the eccentric (lowering) phase — critical for progressing toward full reps with proper form.

How to Perform It

1. Begin in a **full push-up position**: hands shoulder-width apart, body in a straight line from head to heels, core engaged.

2. Slowly **lower your chest toward the ground** over a count of 4–6 seconds, maintaining full-body tension.

3. Stop just before your chest touches the floor, then gently **drop your knees** and reset back to the top position.

4. Repeat for **5–8 slow, controlled reps**, emphasizing quality over quantity.

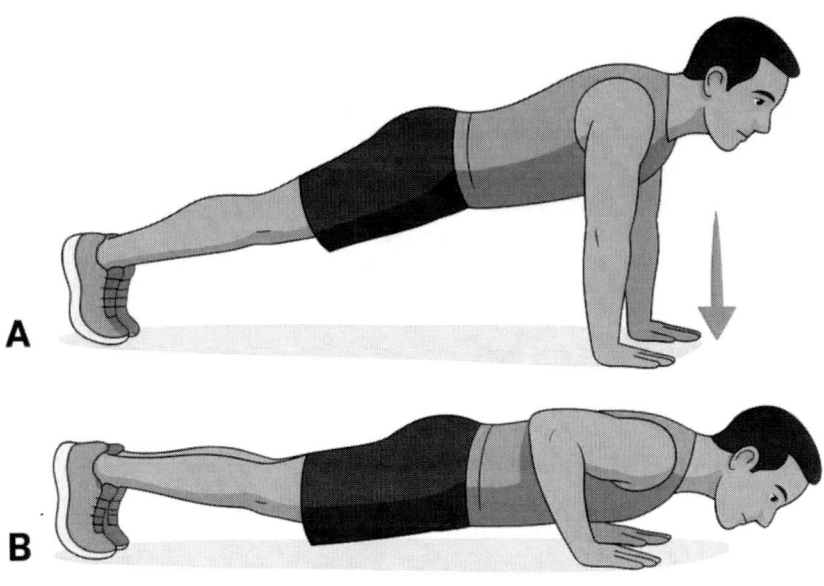

Execution Keys

- Focus on **slow, consistent descent** — fight gravity every inch of the way.

- Maintain a rigid line from your shoulders to heels throughout the lowering phase.

- Keep **elbows at a 45° angle** — avoid flaring out or collapsing.

- Engage your **glutes and abs** for full-body tension.

- Inhale as you lower. No rushing — control is the goal.

⚠ **Safety Tip**

Avoid holding your breath during the descent. If your hips drop faster than your chest, regress to a kneeling negative push-up until you build more control.

Shoulder Taps

Purpose

To improve shoulder stability, core control, and anti-rotation strength while reinforcing proper pushing mechanics in a reduced-load incline position.

How to Perform It

1. Set up in a **high incline plank** with your hands on a stable surface (like a bench or box), feet hip-width apart, and body in a straight line from head to heels.

2. Engage your core and glutes tightly.

3. Lift your **right hand** off the surface and tap your **left shoulder**, keeping your hips and torso as still as possible.

4. Return your right hand to the incline, then repeat with your **left hand** tapping your right shoulder.

5. Continue alternating taps for **10–16 reps total**, moving slowly and with precision.

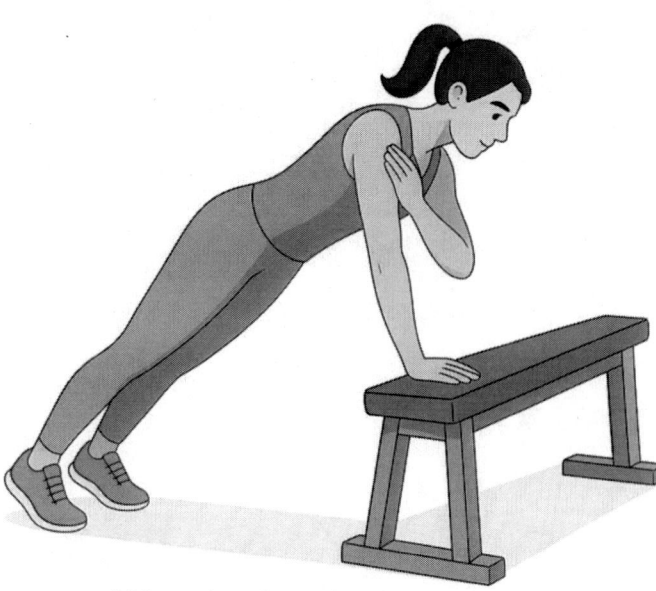

Execution Keys

- Keep **your hips square** — the goal is to avoid rocking or twisting.

- Widen your feet if needed to improve stability.

- Focus on **control, not speed** — slow taps build deeper strength.

- Maintain full tension through your core and glutes the entire time.

- Breathe evenly — no breath holding.

⚠ Safety Tip

Avoid sagging or arching your back during the taps. If form breaks, raise the incline or reduce reps until control improves.

Why It Matters

Inclined shoulder taps challenge your **anti-rotation stability**, one of the most overlooked components in beginner push training. They help condition the scapular stabilizers, teach midline control, and reinforce plank integrity. This movement is not just a core drill — it's a stability benchmark for safe, strong upper body progressions in calisthenics.

Wall Shoulder Push-Up

Purpose

To build foundational overhead pressing strength and shoulder stability while reinforcing scapular control — a key preparation for pike and handstand push-up progressions.

How to Perform It

1. Stand about 2–3 feet away from a wall and place your **hands flat against it** at **eye-level**, slightly wider than shoulder-width.
2. Step your feet back slightly and **hinge at your hips**, so your torso leans forward and your back stays straight — your body should form an inverted "L" shape.
3. Bend your elbows and **lower your head toward the wall**, simulating a vertical press.
4. Stop just before your forehead touches the wall, then press back to the starting position with control.
5. Perform **8–10 controlled reps**, keeping your hips stable and spine neutral.

Execution Keys

- Keep your **elbows at a 45° angle** from your head — not flared out.
- Maintain a **neutral neck** — don't crane forward or look up.
- Press through your palms evenly and **engage your core** to avoid leaning.
- Focus on **vertical movement**, not horizontal push-up mechanics.
- Inhale as you lower; exhale to press up.

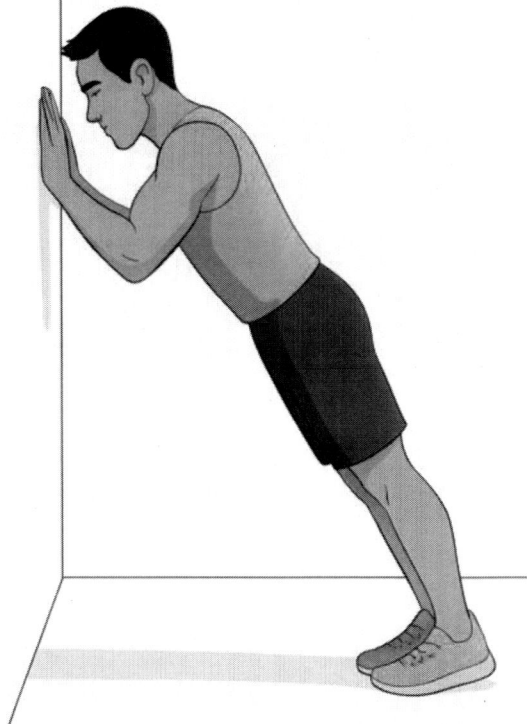

⚠ **Safety Tip**

If your shoulders feel pinched or strained, reduce your range of motion or adjust your hand placement higher on the wall until it feels natural and strong.

Seated Arm Push

Purpose

To activate the triceps, shoulders, and postural muscles through a floor-based pressing movement that reinforces upright torso control without back support.

How to Perform It

1. Sit upright on the floor with your **legs crossed or extended**, spine tall, and **no back support** behind you.
2. Place your **hands flat on the floor** beside your hips, fingertips pointing slightly forward.
3. Engage your core and **press your palms downward** into the floor, as if trying to lift your torso up — but without actually leaving the ground.
4. Hold the **active push** for 3–5 seconds, feeling tension through your triceps and shoulders.
5. Relax briefly, then repeat for **8–10 reps**, maintaining tall posture throughout.

Execution Keys

- Sit as tall as possible — this isn't just about pressing, it's about **postural integrity**.
- Keep your **neck long and shoulders down**, away from your ears.
- Press through the **heel of your palm**, not your fingers.
- Avoid slouching or leaning backward — stay vertical.
- Exhale as you push, inhale as you reset.

⚠ Safety Tip

If wrist pressure becomes uncomfortable, perform the exercise on soft padding or slightly rotate your hands outward to reduce tension.

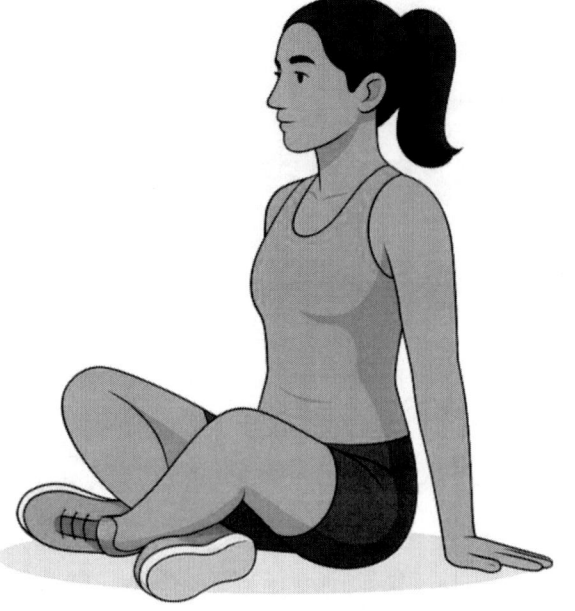

Why It Matters

The seated arm push looks simple, but it's a hidden gem for beginners. It builds **joint awareness**, reinforces **pressing mechanics**, and strengthens the arms and shoulders through active engagement without added load. It's also one of the best tools for correcting rounded shoulders and slumped posture from daily desk habits.

Elevated Pike Push-Up

Purpose

To strengthen the shoulders, triceps, and upper back with vertical pressing mechanics — preparing the body for advanced calisthenics skills like wall-assisted handstand push-ups.

How to Perform It

1. Begin by placing your **feet on a stable elevated surface** (e.g., bench or box) and your **hands on the floor**, shoulder-width apart.
2. Walk your hands back slightly until your body forms an inverted "V" shape — hips high, head between the arms, and legs extended.
3. Bend your elbows and **lower the crown of your head** toward the floor, keeping elbows tucked at a 45° angle.
4. Pause just before your head touches the ground, then press back up to the starting position.
5. Perform **6–10 reps** with control and full-body tension.

Execution Keys

- Keep your **hips stacked over your shoulders** to emphasize vertical loading.
- Do not flare your elbows — maintain **tight press angles**.
- Engage your **core and glutes** to stabilize your body and prevent arching.
- Inhale as you lower, exhale as you press.
- Move in a straight line — **not forward or backward**, just up and down.

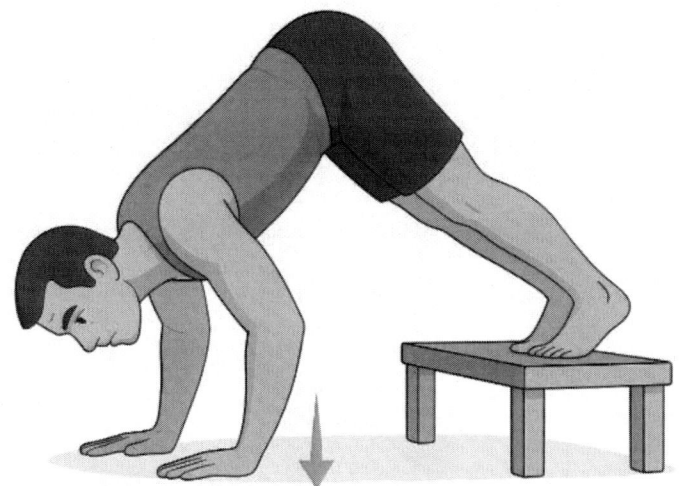

⚠ Safety Tip

If your shoulders feel impinged or unstable, reduce the elevation or perform the movement with your feet on the floor in a standard pike push-up variation.

Why It Matters

The elevated pike push-up bridges the gap between basic shoulder pressing and full handstand variations. It teaches control under vertical load, builds significant upper body strength, and reinforces the alignment necessary for high-skill calisthenics movements. It's a demanding but essential drill in your pushing progression.

Chapter 6: Pull Mechanics Without Equipment

Pull-Based Movements

If push mechanics sculpt the front of the body, **pull mechanics are what hold you upright** — literally. The muscles responsible for posture, scapular control, and back strength are often neglected in bodyweight training simply because true pulling is harder to simulate without equipment. But that doesn't mean it's impossible.

In this chapter, we'll unlock **calisthenics-based pulling exercises that require no bars, straps, or weights** — just gravity, leverage, and intentional movement. These exercises will focus on activating and strengthening the **posterior chain**: your upper back, lats, rhomboids,rear delts, and even grip and forearm stability.

You'll also train **scapular retraction, depression, and stability**, which are essential for long-term shoulder health and balanced muscle development. This chapter is a must for anyone looking to move beyond push-dominant routines and unlock true structural symmetry.

What You'll Gain in This Chapter

- Improved posture and shoulder alignment
- Increased strength in your back and scapular stabilizers
- A foundation for future pulling skills like rows and pull-ups
- Safer, more balanced development across your upper body
- Creative variations that make the most of friction, leverage, and positioning — no gear needed

Just because you don't have a pull-up bar doesn't mean you can't **pull with power**. These next six exercises are proof that where there's intention, there's adaptation — and real strength follows.

Dead Hang

Purpose

To build foundational grip strength, decompress the spine, and activate the lats and shoulders — serving as a crucial entry point to pull-up strength and shoulder health.

How to Perform It

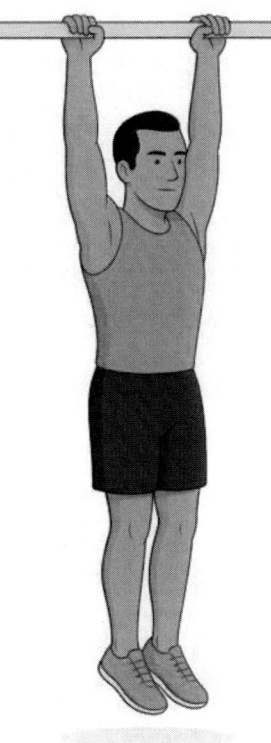

1. Find a sturdy overhead bar, tree limb, or horizontal support that can safely hold your full bodyweight.

2. Jump or step up and grab the bar with an **overhand grip**, hands slightly wider than shoulders.

3. Allow your body to **hang freely**, keeping your legs relaxed and feet off the ground.

4. Gently **engage your lats and core** — don't just dangle — by pulling your shoulders down and away from your ears.

5. Hold the position for **10–30 seconds**, or as long as your grip allows with good form. Lower down gently.

Execution Keys

- Think "**long spine, packed shoulders**" — not loose or slouched.
- Keep your **neck neutral** and breathe steadily.
- Squeeze the bar with your fingers and thumbs to activate grip strength.
- If full hang is too difficult, start with **feet slightly touching** the floor or use a lower bar for partial weight.
- Progressively increase hang time each week.

⚠ Safety Tip

Avoid swinging or rotating under the bar. If your shoulders feel unstable, start with a **scapular-supported dead hang** by gently activating your shoulder blades downward without fully relaxing.

Why It Matters

The dead hang is more than a test of grip — it's a **total upper body primer**. It decompresses the spine, strengthens the lats and forearms, and builds the raw joint integrity required for all pulling movements. For beginners, it's the most accessible way to train pull mechanics before you can perform active pulls or rows.

Doorway Row

Purpose

To develop horizontal pulling strength, improve scapular retraction, and train the back and arms — all using nothing more than a stable doorway and your own bodyweight.

How to Perform It

1. Stand inside a sturdy doorway and grip **both sides of the doorframe** at about chest level. Your feet should be flat and slightly forward, knees bent.

2. Lean back slightly so your arms extend fully, keeping your **body in a straight diagonal line**.

3. From this position, pull your chest toward the frame by **driving your elbows back** and squeezing your shoulder blades together.

4. Pause briefly at the top, then **lower yourself back with control** to the starting position.

5. Perform **8–12 controlled reps**, adjusting foot position to modify difficulty.

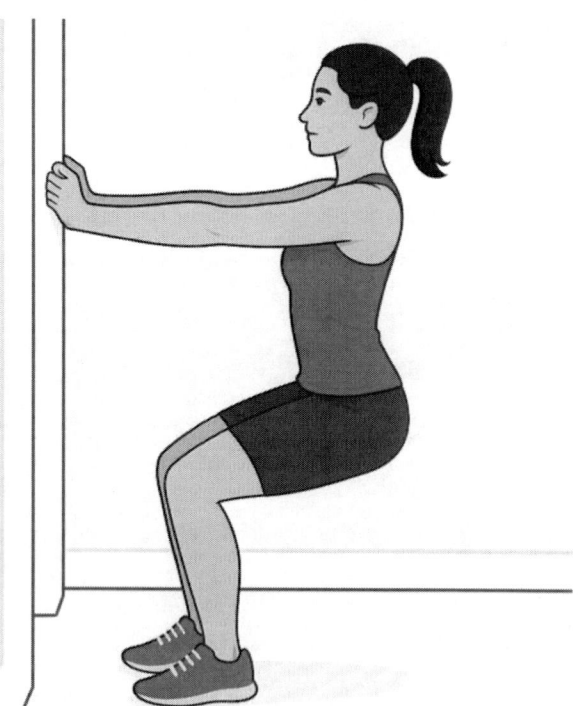

Execution Keys

- Keep your **core braced and spine tall** throughout the pull.
- Think "**pull with the elbows, not the hands**" to maximize back engagement.
- To reduce intensity, **step back** and keep your body more upright.
- To increase difficulty, **walk your feet forward** and lean back further.
- Maintain a smooth rhythm — no jerking or shrugging.

⚠ Safety Tip

Ensure the doorway is **stable and secure**. Avoid pulling with slippery hands or using fragile trim. If in doubt, reinforce the grip area with a towel for friction and comfort.

Towel Pull

Purpose

To simulate the rowing motion and build neuromuscular control in the back, biceps, and scapular stabilizers through isometric contraction — without needing any pull-up bars or weights.

How to Perform It

1. Sit tall and hold a towel with **both hands shoulder-width apart**, as if pulling a rope toward your chest.
2. Extend your arms fully in front of you, then **pull the towel apart slightly** to create outward tension.
3. Begin the rowing motion by **bending your elbows** and drawing the towel toward your upper abdomen.
4. Once in the "rowed" position (hands near chest, elbows pulled behind), **squeeze your shoulder blades together** and hold the contraction for **5–10 seconds**.
5. Release slowly and repeat for **5–8 controlled reps**.

Execution Keys

- Focus on **actively squeezing** your mid-back — not just pulling with your arms.
- Keep your **shoulders down** away from your ears during the hold.
- Generate real tension by **pulling the towel apart** while you row it in.
- Keep your **chest lifted** and posture upright the entire time.

⚠ Safety Tip

If you feel strain in your neck or shoulders, reset your posture and reduce the pulling tension. The motion should feel strong but never forced.

Why It Matters

This movement mimics the mechanics of a row **without needing resistance bands, weights, or a pull-up bar**. The towel acts as a tactile cue to train intent, scapular control, and **isometric pulling strength** — essential for beginners learning how to "feel" their back working before progressing to full-body pulling exercises.

Wall Slides

Purpose

To improve scapular upward rotation, shoulder blade control, and posture — essential for pain-free overhead movement and healthy pulling mechanics.

How to Perform It

1. Stand with your **back flat against a wall**, feet about 6–8 inches away from it, and **lower back gently pressed** into the wall.

2. Raise your arms into a **goalpost position** (elbows bent at 90°, hands near your head), with the **backs of your hands, wrists, and elbows touching the wall** if possible.

3. Slowly **slide your arms upward** along the wall, reaching as high as you can without losing contact or arching your back.

4. Pause briefly at the top, then **slide back down** to the starting position with control.

5. Perform **8–10 slow reps**, focusing on smooth motion and full control.

Execution Keys

- Keep your **core lightly engaged** to maintain a neutral spine.
- Don't force range — only go as high as you can maintain full contact.
- Think "**elbows drive the motion**," not wrists alone.
- Move **slowly** — this is about control, not speed.
- Exhale as you raise, inhale as you lower.

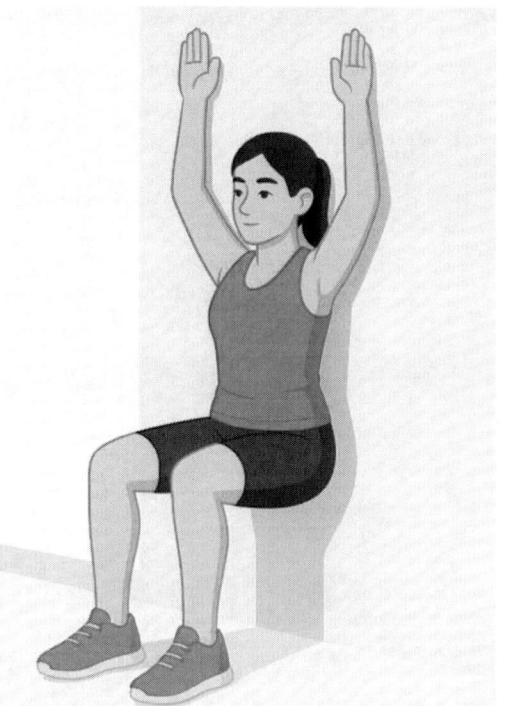

⚠ **Safety Tip**

If your shoulders feel pinched or tight, perform the movement away from the wall or try a floor-based version first until mobility improves.

Why It Matters

Wall slides retrain your shoulders and scapulae to **move in harmony**, improving mobility for overhead lifts and reducing the risk of impingement. For beginners, it's a foundational mobility drill that builds the **postural awareness and control** needed for pain-free calisthenics progressions — especially those involving pull-ups or handstand training.

Reverse Arm Flaps

Purpose

To activate and warm up the rear deltoids, rhomboids, and upper back muscles using dynamic shoulder extension — promoting postural balance and pulling readiness.

How to Perform It

1. Stand tall with your **feet shoulder-width apart** and arms relaxed by your sides.
2. Extend your arms **straight behind you**, palms facing inward or slightly up.
3. Begin making small, **controlled upward pulses** with both arms behind you, squeezing your shoulder blades together.
4. Perform these pulses continuously for **20–30 seconds**, maintaining upright posture and tension.
5. Rest briefly, then repeat for **2–3 rounds** if desired.

Execution Keys

- Keep arms **long and straight** — avoid bending the elbows.
- Focus on **initiating movement from your upper back**, not the arms alone.
- Maintain a **neutral spine and engaged core** to avoid arching.
- Squeeze the **shoulder blades together** on each pulse.
- Breathe naturally and keep the neck relaxed.

⚠ Safety Tip

Avoid arching your lower back to create motion. If you feel shoulder strain, reduce range of motion or lower the arms slightly.

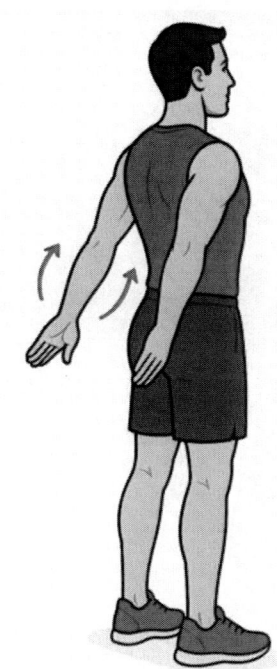

Why It Matters

Reverse arm flaps are deceptively simple but powerful for **activating the upper posterior chain**, a key area often neglected in push-dominant routines. They improve scapular awareness, posture, and muscular endurance — all critical for long-term calisthenics success. This makes them a perfect warm-up or burnout drill in any pulling-focused session.

Wall Pull-Backs

Purpose

To train active scapular retraction and mid-back engagement using only bodyweight and intent — ideal for beginners learning how to "pull" without external resistance.

How to Perform It

1. Stand facing a flat wall, **feet shoulder-width apart**, and knees slightly soft.
2. Reach your arms **straight forward**, palms lightly pressing into the wall at shoulder height.
3. Begin to **pull your elbows backward** in a rowing motion, keeping your hands in contact with the wall as long as possible.
4. As your elbows move past your torso, **squeeze your shoulder blades together** and pause briefly.
5. Return to the starting position with control. Perform **8–12 slow repetitions**.

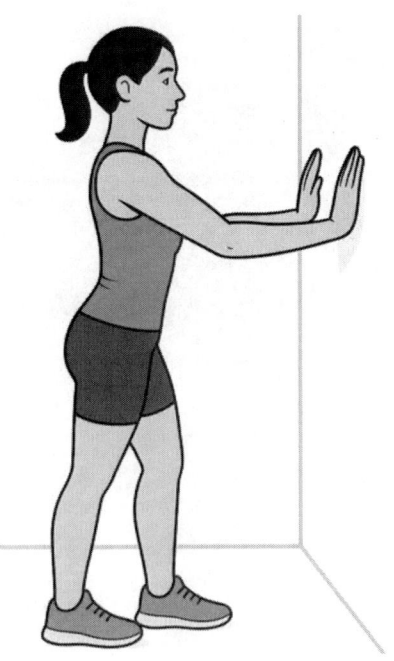

Execution Keys

- Imagine dragging the wall **toward you**, creating internal resistance.
- Keep your **shoulders down and chest lifted** as you pull.
- Don't let your hands lift too soon — **maximize the "slide" back.**
- Lead with your elbows, not your hands.
- Exhale as you pull, inhale as you reset.

⚠ Safety Tip

Do not overreach or lock your elbows at the start. If shoulder discomfort occurs, slightly lower the arm height and reduce wall pressure.

Why It Matters

This resistance-free movement teaches beginners to **actively recruit back muscles**, especially the rhomboids and mid traps, without needing bands or weights. It builds neuromuscular coordination, reinforces posture, and introduces horizontal pulling mechanics — forming the final layer in your foundational pull toolkit.

Chapter 7: Leg Strength & Lower Body Control

Lower Body Exercises

Your legs are the foundation of everything you do — in life and in calisthenics. Whether you're climbing stairs, landing a jump, or holding a strong plank, it all starts from the ground up. But leg training isn't just about squats and brute force. It's about developing **control, symmetry, and functional strength** that supports your full-body mechanics.

In calisthenics, you don't have the luxury of loading a barbell or using machines. You learn to **leverage your own bodyweight**, master angles, and use tempo, positioning, and mobility to extract strength from movement itself. That's why bodyweight leg training builds more than muscle — it builds **awareness, joint integrity, and balance**.

This chapter is designed to train your legs **comprehensively**:

- Glutes, quads, hamstrings, and calves
- Hip stability and ankle mobility
- Unilateral control and structural alignment
- Balance, deceleration, and strength through full range of motion

These aren't just exercises — they're **movement solutions** for real-world function.

What to Expect

You'll start with **bilateral movements** that emphasize stability and range, then progress into **single-leg drills** that build control and expose weaknesses. By the end of this chapter, you'll have the tools to move better, stand stronger, and generate power from the ground up — without touching a weight.

If you've ever skipped leg day before, this chapter changes that permanently.

Bodyweight Squats

Purpose

To build strength and mobility in the quads, glutes, hamstrings, and hips — forming the cornerstone of all lower-body movement patterns in calisthenics.

How to Perform It

1. Stand tall with your **feet shoulder-width apart** and toes slightly turned out.
2. Engage your core, lift your chest, and begin the movement by **pushing your hips back**, then bending your knees to lower into a squat.
3. Keep your **knees aligned with your toes** and your heels grounded throughout.
4. Descend until your thighs are at least parallel to the floor, or as low as mobility allows without rounding your back.
5. Press through your heels to return to standing, squeezing your glutes at the top. Repeat for **10–15 reps**.

Execution Keys

- Keep your **chest lifted** and spine long throughout the movement.
- Focus on **hips back first**, then knees — not the other way around.
- **Drive through your heels**, not your toes, on the way up.
- Use a **slow and controlled tempo**, especially on the descent.
- Arms can extend forward for counterbalance or stay at your chest.

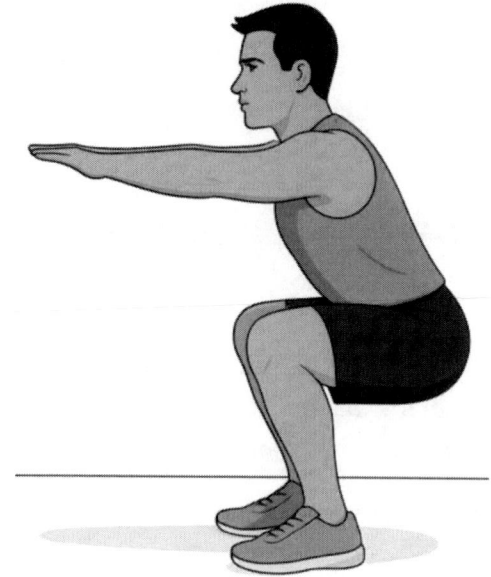

⚠ Safety Tip

Avoid letting your **knees collapse inward** or your **heels lift off the floor**. If your mobility is limited, start with a **box or chair behind you** for support and depth control.

Step-Back Lunges

Purpose

To strengthen the quads, hamstrings, and glutes while improving single-leg balance, coordination, and control — essential for calisthenics leg progression.

How to Perform It

1. Stand tall with your **feet hip-width apart** and arms at your sides or on your hips.
2. Shift your weight slightly onto your left foot, then **step your right foot back** about 2–3 feet.
3. Lower your body by **bending both knees** until your front thigh is parallel to the floor and your back knee hovers just above the ground.
4. Press through your **front heel** to rise back up and return to standing.
5. Alternate sides and perform **8–10 reps per leg**.

Execution Keys

- Keep your **torso upright** — avoid leaning forward.
- Your **front knee** should stay aligned over your ankle, not past your toes.
- Keep your **core engaged** to maintain balance.
- Step straight back — avoid crossing behind the body.
- Inhale as you lower, exhale as you drive up.

⚠ Safety Tip

If you experience knee discomfort, **reduce your range of motion** and keep your step shorter. Always ensure that your front heel stays fully grounded.

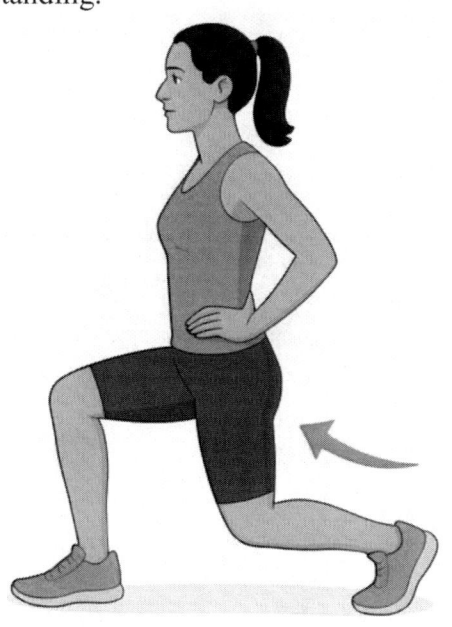

Why It Matters

Step-back lunges are a controlled, joint-friendly way to develop single-leg strength without putting excess stress on the knees. They enhance balance, spatial awareness, and glute engagement — all of which are crucial for more advanced skills like pistol squats, jump variations, and explosive power work. They're a key transition from bilateral to unilateral leg mastery in calisthenics.

Wall Sit

Purpose

To develop lower body endurance, isometric strength, and mental grit by maintaining a static squat position — ideal for joint stabilization and muscular conditioning.

How to Perform It

1. Stand with your **back flat against a wall**, feet shoulder-width apart and about **two feet away** from the wall.

2. Slide down the wall until your **knees are bent at a 90° angle** and your thighs are parallel to the floor.

3. Keep your **knees aligned over your ankles**, not extending past your toes.

4. Hold this position for **30–60 seconds**, or as long as form can be maintained.

5. Slowly press yourself back up the wall to return to standing. Rest and repeat for **2–3 rounds** if desired.

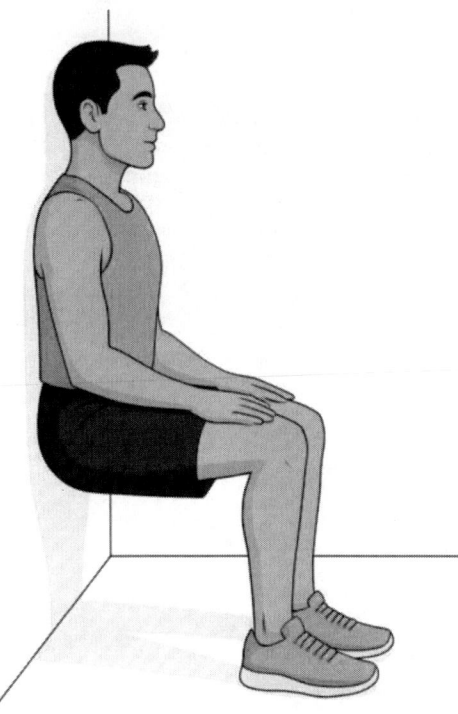

Execution Keys

- Keep your **lower back and shoulders in contact** with the wall.

- Distribute your weight **evenly through both feet**, pressing firmly into the floor.

- Keep your **head neutral** and your gaze forward — avoid tensing the neck.

- Engage your **core and glutes** to stabilize the hold.

⚠ Safety Tip

Avoid letting your **knees drift inward** or your back arch off the wall. If you feel joint pressure instead of muscle engagement, reduce depth or adjust foot position.

Why It Matters

The wall sit is a powerful isometric drill that builds **quadriceps endurance, mental resilience, and postural discipline**. It teaches you how to maintain tension under fatigue — a skill that directly translates to static holds, advanced calisthenics skills, and everyday functional strength. It's simple, scalable, and brutally effective.

Glute Bridge March

Purpose

To strengthen the glutes, hamstrings, and deep core muscles while reinforcing pelvic stability through unilateral movement from a supported position.

How to Perform It

1. Lie on your back with your **knees bent**, feet flat on the floor, and arms extended by your sides, palms down.
2. Engage your core and glutes, then lift your hips into a **bridge position**, forming a straight line from shoulders to knees.
3. Without letting your hips drop, **lift your right foot off the ground**, bringing the knee toward your chest.
4. Lower the foot back down with control, then **repeat on the left side** — alternating in a slow, marching rhythm.
5. Perform **6–8 marches per leg**, maintaining tension throughout.

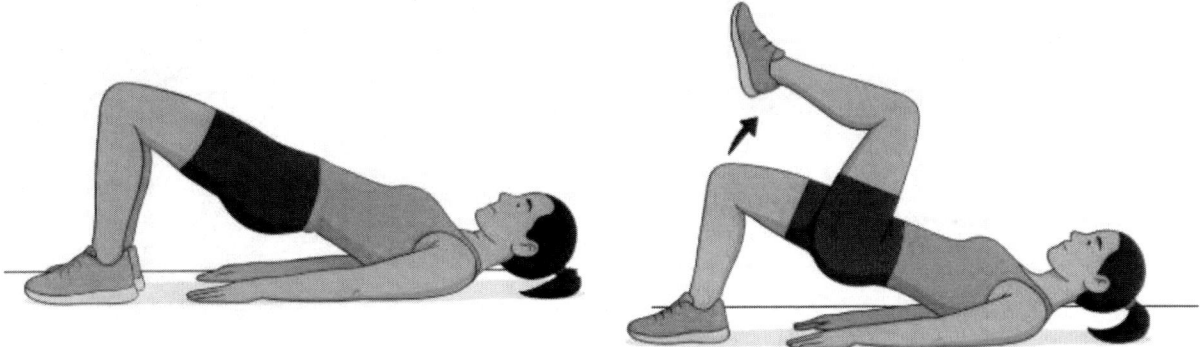

Execution Keys

- Keep your **hips level** as you lift each leg — avoid wobbling or dropping.
- Drive down through the **heel of the supporting foot**.
- Focus on **slow, controlled movement**, not speed.
- Brace your **core** and avoid overarching the lower back.

⚠ Safety Tip

If your lower back begins to tense or arch, lower your hips slightly or reduce march height. Focus on **glute activation**, not lumbar compensation.

Lateral Step-Over

Purpose

To develop lateral hip strength, balance, and coordination by stepping side-to-side over a low object — enhancing functional movement and pelvic control.

How to Perform It

1. Stand upright next to a **low, stable object** (like a yoga block, step, or small cone), feet together.

2. Shift your weight onto your inside leg and **lift the outside leg**, stepping laterally over the object.

3. Gently **plant the lifted foot on the other side**, then bring the second foot across to return to a neutral stance.

4. Immediately **step back in the opposite direction**, repeating the sequence back and forth.

5. Perform **8–10 step-overs per direction**, maintaining rhythm and posture.

Execution Keys

- Choose an object that allows a **controlled step**, not a jump.
- Keep your **chest upright and gaze forward** — avoid looking down.
- Engage your **core and hips** to maintain balance during the transition.
- Land each step with a **soft, deliberate motion** — no stomping.
- Use arms for light counterbalance if needed.

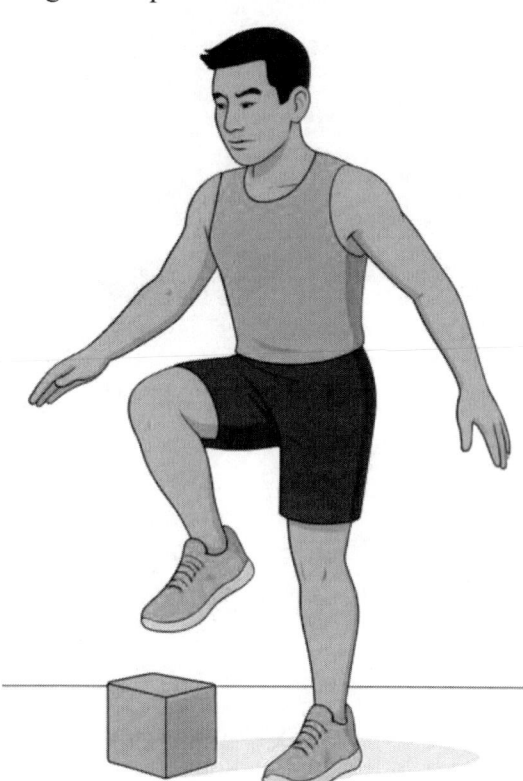

⚠ Safety Tip

Avoid lifting your leg excessively high or rushing the movement. If you lose balance frequently, **reduce the object height** or step without an object to build confidence first.

Calf Raise Hold

Purpose

To build strength and endurance in the calves, ankles, and foot stabilizers while enhancing balance and joint support through isometric contraction.

How to Perform It

1. Stand tall with your **feet hip-width apart**, arms relaxed at your sides or lightly touching a wall for balance.
2. Slowly rise onto the **balls of your feet**, lifting your heels as high as possible.
3. Engage your calves and **hold the top position** for **10–20 seconds** without bouncing.
4. Lower your heels back down with control.
5. Rest briefly and repeat for **2–3 rounds**.

Execution Keys

- Press evenly through the **base of your big toe and pinky toe** — avoid rolling outward.
- Keep your **legs straight but not locked**.
- Focus on lifting through the **center of the body**, maintaining tall posture.
- Breathe steadily — avoid holding your breath.
- Use a mirror or tactile cue (like fingertips on a wall) to monitor balance.

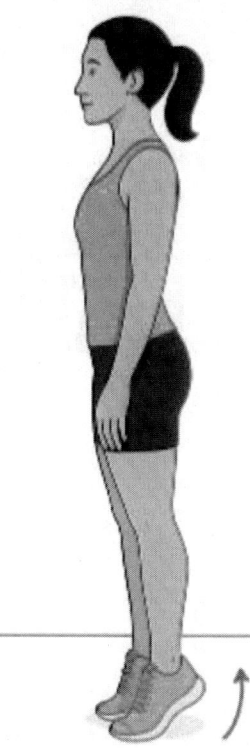

⚠ Safety Tip

If you experience cramping or instability, **shorten the hold time** and reduce height slightly. Progress only as stability and control improve.

Why It Matters

Often overlooked, your calves and ankles are the final link in your lower-body kinetic chain. Strong calves mean **better balance, stronger jumps, improved posture, and safer landings** — all key in bodyweight training. The isometric hold builds muscular endurance and joint integrity that carries over into almost every movement you perform, from squats to sprinting.

Kneeling Hip Extension

Purpose

To isolate and strengthen the gluteus maximus while reinforcing hip extension mechanics — critical for building power, stability, and control in calisthenics leg movements.

How to Perform It

1. Begin on all fours in a **quadruped position**, with your hands under your shoulders and knees under your hips.

2. Keeping your core tight and spine neutral, **lift your right leg** by driving the heel upward toward the ceiling, keeping the knee bent at 90°.

3. Pause briefly at the top when your **thigh aligns with your torso**, then slowly lower back to start.

4. Repeat for **10–12 reps**, then switch to the left side.

5. Maintain steady breathing and avoid twisting your hips.

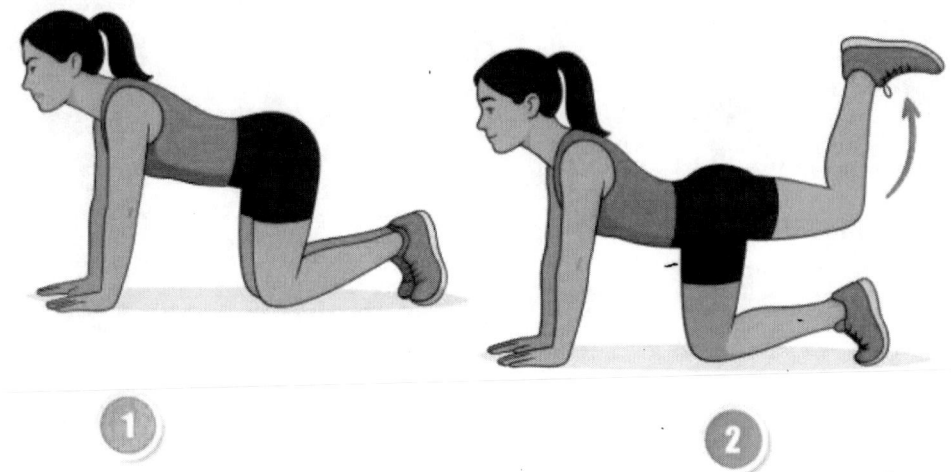

Execution Keys

- Keep your **hips square** — avoid rotating or leaning.
- Drive the movement from your **glute**, not your lower back.
- Maintain a **neutral spine** and engaged core throughout.
- Press your **heel up and back**, not your toe.

⚠ Safety Tip

If you feel strain in your lower back, reduce your range of motion and refocus on glute engagement. The lift should come from **hip extension**, not spinal movement.

Supported Pistol Prep

Purpose

To build the strength, balance, and joint control needed for full pistol squats by using external support to safely rehearse the single-leg pattern.

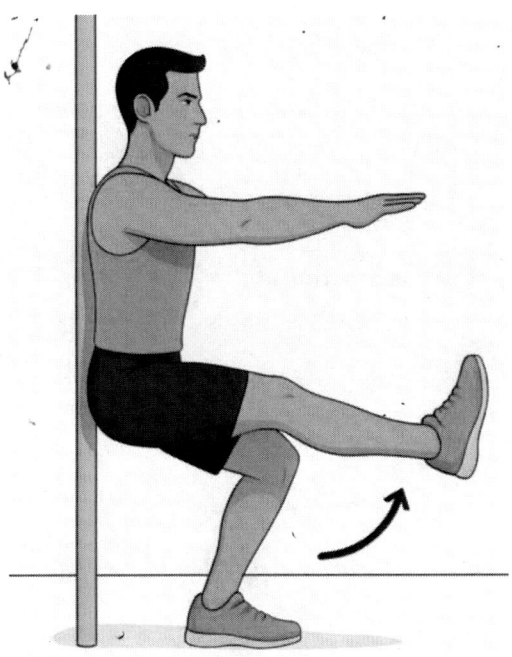

How to Perform It

1. Stand in front of a **box, bench, or sturdy pole** with feet hip-width apart.

2. Shift your weight onto your **left leg** while holding lightly onto the support.

3. Extend your **right leg forward**, keeping it straight and hovering above the ground.

4. Begin to **lower yourself slowly** into a squat on your left leg, using the support only as needed for balance and control.

5. Lower to the box (if using one) or as low as mobility allows, then press through your right heel to return to standing.

6. Perform **5–8 reps per leg**, alternating sides.

Execution Keys

- Keep your **chest upright** and eyes forward — don't collapse the torso.
- **Drive through the heel** of the standing leg, not the toes.
- Use the support only for **stability, not leverage**.
- **Extend the free leg** fully to counterbalance the motion.

⚠ Safety Tip

Avoid forcing the depth. If your **knee caves inward** or you feel strain in your hips, **reduce range of motion** or increase box height. Never "fall" into the bottom of the movement.

Why It Matters

The pistol squat is a signature calisthenics skill — but jumping into it unprepared is a recipe for frustration or injury. This supported variation builds **confidence, mobility, and foundational control**. It trains unilateral strength while protecting the joints and teaches your nervous system how to manage your full bodyweight on one leg — an essential stepping stone to mastering advanced leg mechanics.

Chair Sit-Down/Stand-Up

Purpose

To develop lower body strength, control, and confidence in a functional movement pattern that mimics squatting — perfect for beginners building mobility and coordination.

How to Perform It

1. Stand in front of a **sturdy chair**, feet about shoulder-width apart, with the back of your legs lightly touching the seat.
2. Cross your arms in front of your chest or hold them out for balance.
3. Slowly **hinge at the hips** and bend your knees to **sit down onto the chair with control**, keeping your torso upright.
4. Pause briefly, then **press through your heels** to stand back up without using your hands.
5. Perform **10–12 repetitions**, focusing on steady movement and posture.

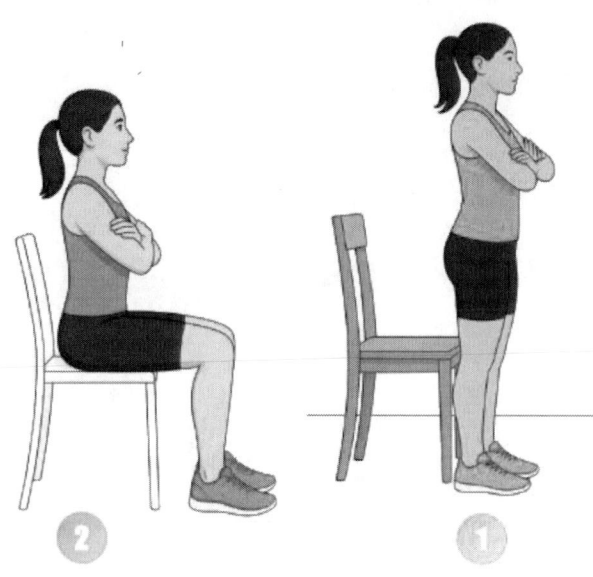

Execution Keys

- Keep your **knees in line with your toes**, not caving inward.
- Engage your **core and glutes** throughout the entire motion.
- Lower with control — don't drop onto the chair.
- Use your **breath to guide the rhythm**: inhale to lower, exhale to rise.
- Position the chair so it's at a comfortable, **knee-height level**.

⚠ **Safety Tip**

If you struggle to stand without momentum, use a slightly **higher chair** or add cushions. Avoid using your arms to push off unless absolutely necessary — the goal is to build **leg strength independently**.

Why It Matters

The chair sit-down/stand-up drill is deceptively powerful. It teaches the **fundamentals of squatting**, hip hinging, and controlled descent — without intimidating depth or complexity.

Single-Leg Reach

Purpose

To challenge lower-body coordination, balance, and glute-hamstring strength by reaching forward while standing on one leg — enhancing joint control and unilateral stability.

How to Perform It

1. Stand tall with your **feet together**, arms relaxed at your sides.
2. Shift your weight onto your **left leg**, lifting your **right foot slightly** off the ground behind you.
3. With your **core engaged**, slowly **hinge at the hips** and reach both hands forward as your lifted leg extends straight behind you.
4. Keep your spine neutral and hips square as you reach as far as balance allows.
5. Return to standing with control. Perform **6–8 reps**, then switch sides.

Execution Keys

- Maintain a **soft bend in the standing leg** — don't lock the knee.
- Focus your gaze on a **fixed point ahead** to help maintain balance.
- Move slowly — this is about **control, not speed**.
- Engage your **core and glutes** throughout the movement.
- Keep your **hips level** — avoid rotating open.

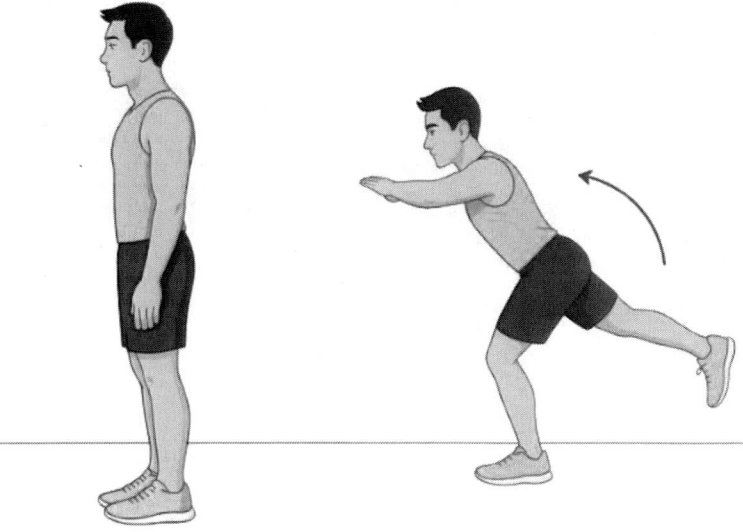

⚠ Safety Tip

Use a wall or chair for light support if your balance is unsteady at first. Avoid reaching so far that it causes **spinal rounding or hip twist**.

Why It Matters

This drill goes beyond strength — it builds **body awareness and control on a single leg**, which is key for injury prevention and advanced movements like pistol squats and jumping transitions. The single-leg reach improves **ankle stability, glute activation, and postural endurance**, making it a smart addition for both beginners and progressing athletes.

Chapter 8: Balance, Coordination & Functional Flow

Stability-Based Movements

Most people train for strength, some for flexibility—but few give enough attention to the connective thread between them: **balance and coordination**. Without these, even the strongest body lacks control, and the most flexible one wobbles in motion. Calisthenics doesn't just reward stability—it demands it.

In this chapter, we turn the spotlight on the **neuromuscular connection**—your body's ability to sense, stabilize, and adjust in real time. These movements may look simple on the surface, but their power lies in teaching your body how to move with quiet precision, deliberate timing, and internal focus.

Whether you're stepping over obstacles, holding your body still in space, or transferring weight from one side to the other, each drill in this section develops your **joint integrity, ankle stability, core integration, and reaction control**—traits that set apart a beginner from a truly functional mover.

You won't need fancy equipment. You won't even need speed. But you will need focus, patience, and control. The exercises ahead build **proprioception** (your body's awareness of its position), helping you feel more connected, centered, and grounded in every movement—on the mat or in everyday life.

By the end of this chapter, you'll walk taller, move smarter, and feel the kind of internal strength that doesn't just show—it *stays*. Let's make your body intelligent, not just strong.

Single-Leg Hold

Purpose

To improve proprioception, core control, and lower-limb stability by removing visual input—challenging your balance through deeper sensory pathways.

How to Perform It

1. Stand tall with your **feet hip-width apart**, arms relaxed at your sides.
2. Shift your weight onto your **right foot**, then gently lift your **left knee to hip height** (or as high as comfortable).
3. Once stable, slowly **close your eyes** and begin timing the hold.
4. Maintain balance for **10–20 seconds**, then lower the leg and switch sides.
5. Perform **2 rounds per side**, keeping your breath calm and even.

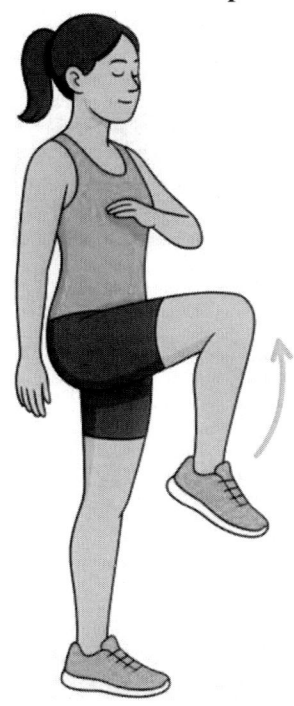

Execution Keys

- Stand near a wall or chair for **safety support** if needed.
- Keep your **core gently braced** to prevent swaying.
- Avoid gripping your toes—**distribute weight evenly** through the standing foot.
- Stay upright — don't lean back or hunch forward.
- Start with **eyes open**, then progress to closed only when steady.

⚠ Safety Tip

Perform this exercise in a **clear, open space** free of obstacles. Use light finger contact on a surface when beginning — avoid doing it unsupervised if your balance is highly unsteady.

Why It Matters

Closing your eyes forces your body to rely on **vestibular and muscular feedback**, not just sight. This unlocks deeper balance coordination and body awareness. It's a powerful, low-impact tool to **train the nervous system, prevent falls, and build true functional control**—especially for beginners, seniors, or anyone returning from injury.

Bear Crawl Walkout

Purpose

To build integrated core strength, shoulder stability, and coordination by transitioning in and out of a bear crawl position with controlled movement.

How to Perform It

1. Begin in a **standing position**, feet hip-width apart, arms at your sides.
2. **Hinge at your hips** and lower your hands to the floor, bending your knees as needed.
3. Step your hands **forward one at a time**, lowering into a **bear crawl position** — knees hover just an inch above the ground, under hips.
4. Hold briefly, keeping your **back flat and core tight**, then **walk your hands back** to your feet.
5. Return to standing with control. Repeat for **6–8 slow walkouts**.

Execution Keys

- Keep your **knees low** and hips in line with shoulders during the bear hold.
- Engage your **core and lats** throughout the walkout and return.
- Avoid **arching the lower back** — maintain a strong, neutral spine.
- Move slowly — this is about **precision, not speed**.

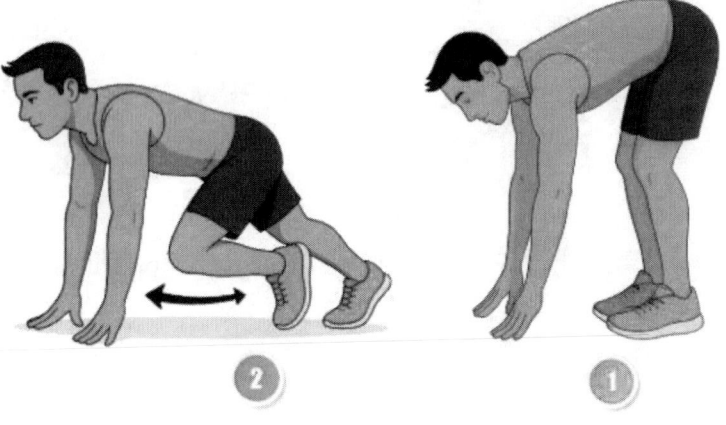

⚠ Safety Tip

Do not let your **hips sag or pike** during the bear crawl hold. Keep movements deliberate and avoid rushing the return to standing — this keeps joints protected and posture intact.

Why It Matters

The bear crawl walkout is a total-body activation drill. It teaches you how to **control your limbs under tension**, reinforces **quadruped stability**, and improves the transition between grounded and upright movements. For calisthenics, this lays the groundwork for crawling patterns, planche variations, and dynamic floor-based strength — all while sharpening coordination and core integration.

Wall-Assisted Handstand Hold

Purpose

To develop shoulder endurance, core control, and full-body alignment while getting comfortable supporting your own bodyweight in an inverted position.

How to Perform It

1. Begin in a **standing position facing away from a wall**, about one leg-length in front of it.
2. **Place your hands on the floor**, shoulder-width apart, about 6–8 inches from the wall.
3. Step one foot up the wall, followed by the other, until your body is in a **straight, vertical line**. Your heels should rest gently on the wall.
4. **Engage your core, squeeze your glutes**, and press strongly through your shoulders to lift up out of the joints.
5. Hold the position for **10–30 seconds**, then carefully come down one foot at a time.

Execution Keys

- Keep your **arms straight** and shoulders elevated — don't sink into the sockets.
- Point your **toes and tighten your quads** for full-body tension.
- Keep your **gaze between your hands** to maintain neck neutrality.
- Your **heels should barely touch** the wall — use it only for balance, not support.
- Progressively increase hold time as strength and control improve.

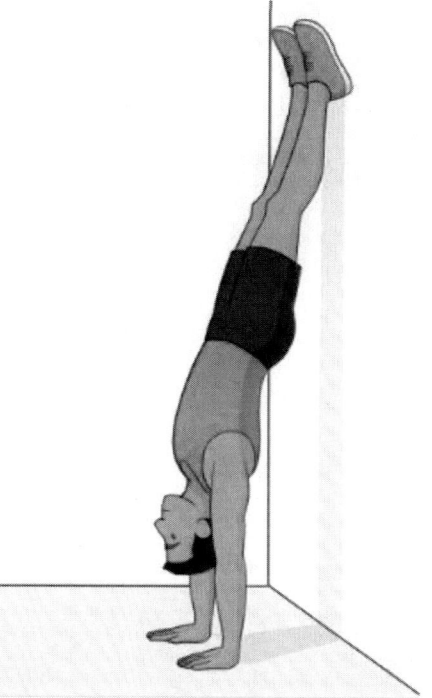

⚠ Safety Tip

Always **practice on a soft surface or mat** and clear the surrounding area. If you feel yourself falling, **tuck and roll out sideways** rather than collapsing forward.

Why It Matters

The wall-assisted handstand hold builds **vertical strength and proprioception**, key traits for calisthenics mastery. It improves shoulder stacking, teaches the body how to **engage under load**, and rewires your sense of balance while upside down. It's also a major confidence builder — proving to yourself that you're capable of holding your own weight in space.

Dynamic March-in-Place

Purpose

To improve rhythm, posture, and dynamic coordination by driving one knee at a time toward the chest with controlled tempo—building full-body awareness without high impact.

How to Perform It

1. Stand tall with your **feet hip-width apart**, arms relaxed at your sides.
2. Engage your core and begin to **lift your right knee** toward hip height as you raise your **left arm** (opposite limb drive).
3. Lower the leg with control and immediately **lift the left knee**, raising the right arm in sync.
4. Continue alternating legs in a **slow, rhythmic march**, focusing on upright posture and muscle control.
5. Perform for **30–45 seconds**, aiming for clean, fluid movement—not speed.

Execution Keys

- Keep your **shoulders relaxed** and chest proud—don't hunch forward.
- Drive your **knees up** rather than pulling them with momentum.
- Engage your **core and glutes** with each lift to maintain balance.
- Land softly on the balls of your feet — avoid stomping.
- Use your **arms actively** to train cross-body movement patterns.

⚠ **Safety Tip**

If balance is an issue, perform the drill next to a **wall or countertop** for support. Avoid leaning back as the knees rise—this puts stress on the lower spine.

Why It Matters

This marching variation improves **neuromuscular timing, dynamic posture, and movement symmetry**. It's perfect for warming up the hips, knees, and spine while also refining the cross-body coordination needed in more complex patterns like crawling, sprinting, or climbing. For beginners, it builds safe movement confidence—one controlled step at a time.

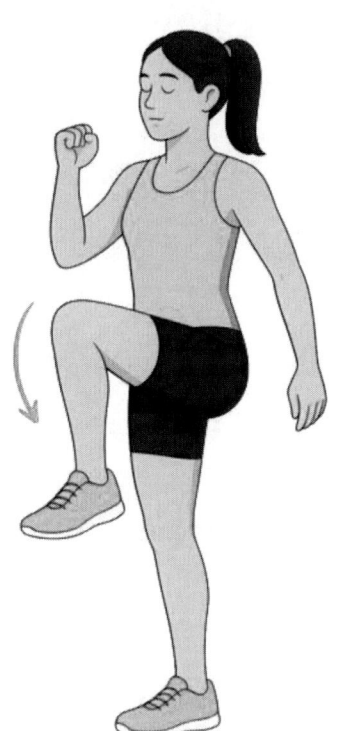

Lateral Crawl Step

Purpose

To develop lateral body control, core engagement, and shoulder stability by moving side-to-side in a low, quadruped position—building dynamic strength and coordination.

How to Perform It

1. Begin in an **all-fours position** with your hands under shoulders and knees under hips.
2. **Lift your knees an inch off the floor**, entering a bear crawl stance—hips low, back flat.
3. Step your **right hand and right foot** to the right simultaneously, followed by the **left hand and left foot**.
4. Move 3–4 steps to the right, pause, then return to the left the same way.
5. Perform for **2 rounds of 4–6 controlled steps each direction**.

Execution Keys

- Maintain a **neutral spine** and low hip height throughout.
- Keep your **knees close to the floor**, not lifted high.
- Move **slowly and deliberately** — avoid bouncing or twisting.
- Engage your **core and shoulder girdle** for control and alignment.
- Keep your **head aligned with your spine**, eyes on the floor.

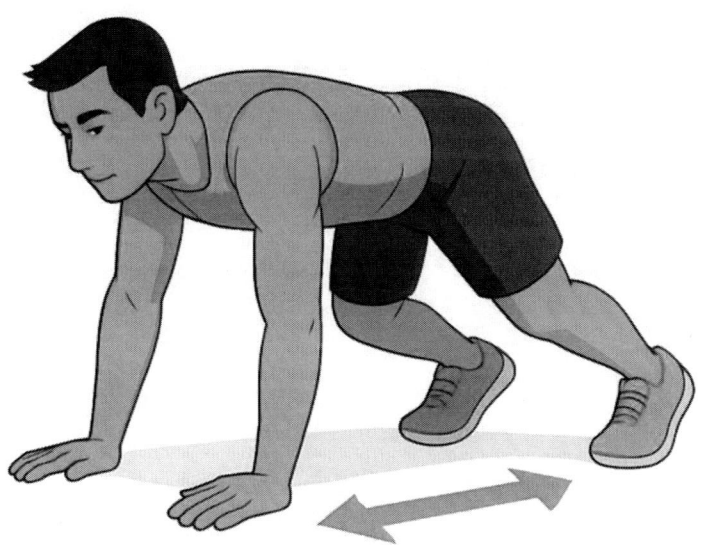

⚠ Safety Tip

If your wrists feel strained, **shift some weight back toward your hips** and limit your range of motion. Avoid sagging your hips or letting your back arch excessively.

Why It Matters

Lateral crawl steps reinforce **multi-limb coordination**, horizontal core tension, and shoulder resilience under load. Unlike standard bear crawls, they train **side-to-side body control**, which is essential for real-world agility, injury prevention, and movement fluency. This variation challenges both stability and awareness—two pillars of functional calisthenics.

Chapter 9: Flexibility & Cooldown Reset

Restore, lengthen, and improve recovery.
Flexibility Sequences (6)

Strength isn't fully realized without flexibility—and mobility is meaningless without recovery. That's why this chapter isn't optional; it's essential. After every push, every crawl, every rep that challenges your structure, your body needs space to **reset, realign, and restore**. That's where flexibility comes in—not just as a cooldown, but as a conscious practice of longevity.

This chapter focuses on **functional stretching**—movements that promote tissue lengthening, joint decompression, and mind-body recalibration. Unlike static "hold and hope" stretches, these sequences are active, mindful, and geared toward improving **circulation, posture, and joint range of motion** over time.

You'll reconnect with your breath, ease muscular tension, and **reduce residual tightness** that accumulates during training. More importantly, you'll train your nervous system to associate movement with control—not threat—which accelerates recovery and keeps your performance consistent.

Each flexibility sequence in this section was chosen not for complexity, but for effectiveness. You don't need to be "bendy." You just need to be present. Whether you're training for strength or simply trying to feel good in your body again, these drills are the missing link between effort and ease.

The better you treat your body in cooldown, the more it will show up for you when it's time to perform again. Let's close strong—with intention, not exhaustion.

Standing Forward Fold

Purpose

To gently lengthen the hamstrings, calves, and lower back while decompressing the spine—promoting calm, flexibility, and postural reset after training.

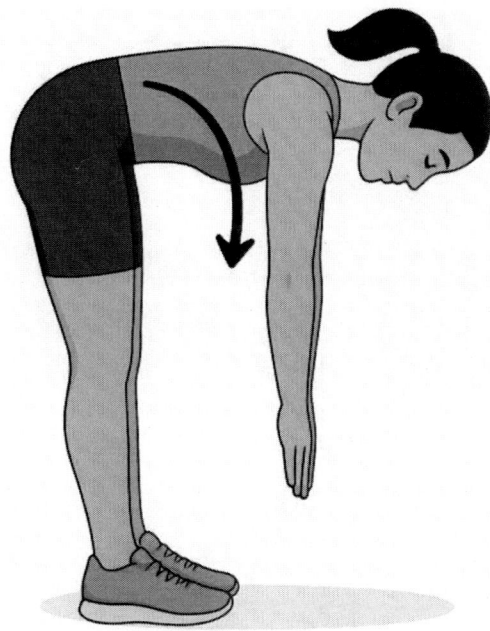

How to Perform It

1. Stand tall with your **feet hip-width apart** and arms resting at your sides.

2. Inhale deeply, then as you **exhale**, hinge at your hips and slowly fold forward—**reaching your hands toward the floor**.

3. Allow your **knees to bend slightly** if your hamstrings feel tight; let your **head hang heavy**.

4. Stay in the fold for **20–30 seconds**, breathing deeply and feeling your spine lengthen.

5. To rise, **bend your knees more deeply**, engage your core, and **roll up slowly** to standing.

Execution Keys

- Keep the **weight centered over your feet**, not on your heels.
- Let your **arms hang or lightly touch the floor/shins**—don't force the reach.
- Use the **breath to deepen the stretch** gently with each exhale.
- Avoid pulling yourself down—this is about release, not reach.
- Focus on **hinging at the hips**, not rounding from the lower back.

⚠ **Safety Tip**

If you feel dizzy when coming up, pause at the bottom and **rise slowly**, supporting yourself with your hands on your thighs if needed. Always avoid bouncing or jerking.

Why It Matters

The standing forward fold is a foundational cool down movement. It encourages **spinal decompression, nervous system calm, and posterior chain release**. After intense bodyweight work, it resets your posture, relieves tension, and reinforces the importance of recovery in any sustainable training program.

Kneeling Hip Flexor Stretch

Purpose

To release tightness in the hip flexors and quads—restoring pelvic alignment, improving stride mechanics, and enhancing recovery after lower-body or core training.

How to Perform It

1. Begin in a **kneeling lunge position** with your right foot forward and left knee resting comfortably on the floor or a mat.
2. Keep your **torso upright**, hands resting on your front thigh for balance.
3. Gently **shift your weight forward** until you feel a stretch along the **front of your left hip**.
4. Squeeze your **left glute** to deepen the stretch and prevent over-arching the lower back.
5. Hold for **20–30 seconds**, then switch legs and repeat on the other side.

Execution Keys

- Keep your **hips squared** forward—avoid twisting or leaning to one side.
- Engage your **glutes and abs** to stabilize the pelvis.
- Keep your **chest lifted** and avoid collapsing into the lower back.
- For added stretch, raise the arm on the **same side as the rear leg** and gently reach overhead.

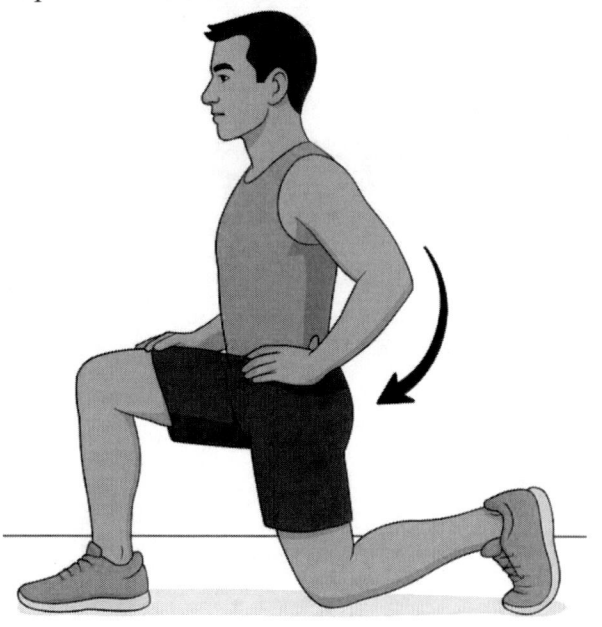

⚠ **Safety Tip**

Avoid **pushing aggressively** into the stretch—especially if you feel tension in the knee. Use a folded towel or pad under the back knee for support if needed.

Why It Matters

Tight hip flexors are one of the most common mobility restrictions—especially in people who sit frequently or perform repetitive forward movements. This stretch restores **front-hip length, pelvic control, and stride efficiency**, making it a vital cooldown for anyone focused on sustainable strength and balance.

Reclined Twist

Purpose

To promote spinal mobility, relieve tension in the lower back and obliques, and enhance recovery through gentle rotation and breath awareness.

How to Perform It

1. Lie on your back with your **arms extended out to the sides** in a T position, palms facing up.
2. Bring both knees up toward your chest, then **let them slowly fall to the right**, keeping your shoulders grounded.
3. Turn your **head to the left** if comfortable, maintaining a long spine.
4. Breathe deeply and hold the stretch for **30–45 seconds**, feeling the twist through your midsection.
5. Gently bring your knees back to center and repeat on the **left side**.

Execution Keys

- Keep both **shoulder blades in contact with the floor**—don't let one peel up.
- Allow the knees to **rest wherever comfortable**, using a pillow or block if needed.
- Use your **breath to guide the stretch**, deepening with each exhale.
- Avoid forcing the twist—this is about release, not intensity.

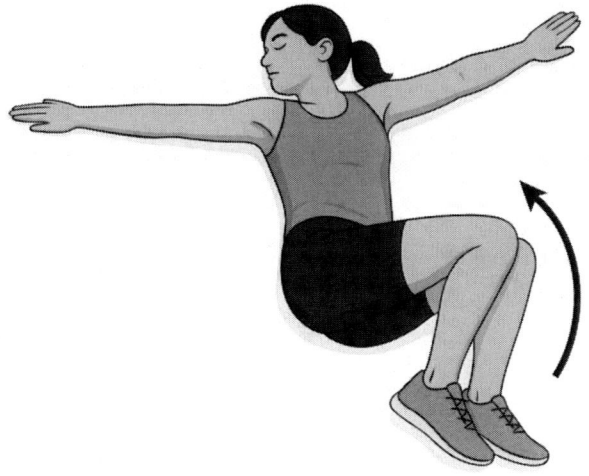

⚠ Safety Tip

If you feel strain in your lower back, reduce the depth of the twist by **placing a cushion under your knees**. Never yank or push the legs down forcefully.

Why It Matters

The reclined twist encourages **spinal decompression, digestive stimulation, and nervous system downregulation**. It's especially effective after workouts that involve rotation, bending, or heavy core engagement. This movement helps the body unwind—literally—leaving you grounded, realigned, and more mobile.

Seated Hamstring Fold

Purpose

To lengthen the hamstrings, release the lower back, and decompress the spine—supporting postural reset and muscular recovery after training.

How to Perform It

1. Sit on the floor with your **legs extended straight out** in front of you, feet flexed and spine tall.
2. Inhale to lengthen your torso, then **exhale and slowly hinge forward** from the hips, reaching toward your toes.
3. Keep your **back flat** as you fold, stopping when you feel a comfortable stretch in the backs of your legs.
4. Rest your hands on your shins, ankles, or feet—whichever feels natural.
5. Hold for **30–45 seconds**, breathing deeply and letting the stretch deepen gently with each exhale.

Execution Keys

- Avoid rounding your upper back—**lead the movement from your hips**.
- Keep your **knees softly bent** if your hamstrings are tight.
- Engage your **quadriceps** to support hamstring lengthening.
- Let your **neck stay neutral**, not straining upward or downward.

⚠ Safety Tip

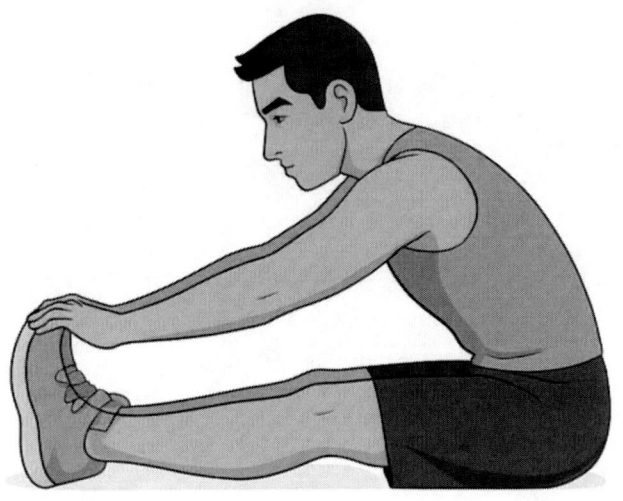

If you feel sharp pulling behind the knees or lower back, **ease out slightly** or elevate your hips by sitting on a folded towel to reduce tension.

Why It Matters

This seated fold is a classic cooldown stretch for good reason—it promotes **hamstring flexibility, posterior chain relief, and spinal decompression**. After standing, walking, squatting, or balancing drills, this movement resets the system and supports **long-term mobility and muscular balance**.

Cobra to Child's Pose Flow

Purpose

To combine gentle spinal extension and flexion into a restorative flow that improves mobility, calms the nervous system, and supports deep recovery post-workout.

How to Perform It

1. Start lying face down, hands placed under your shoulders, elbows tucked in.
2. Press into your palms and gently **lift your chest into a low cobra pose**, keeping your pelvis grounded and shoulders relaxed.
3. Inhale in cobra, then **exhale as you push back into child's pose**—hips to heels, arms extended forward.
4. Pause in child's pose for a breath or two, then **flow back to cobra**.
5. Repeat this fluid transition for **4–6 slow, intentional rounds**.

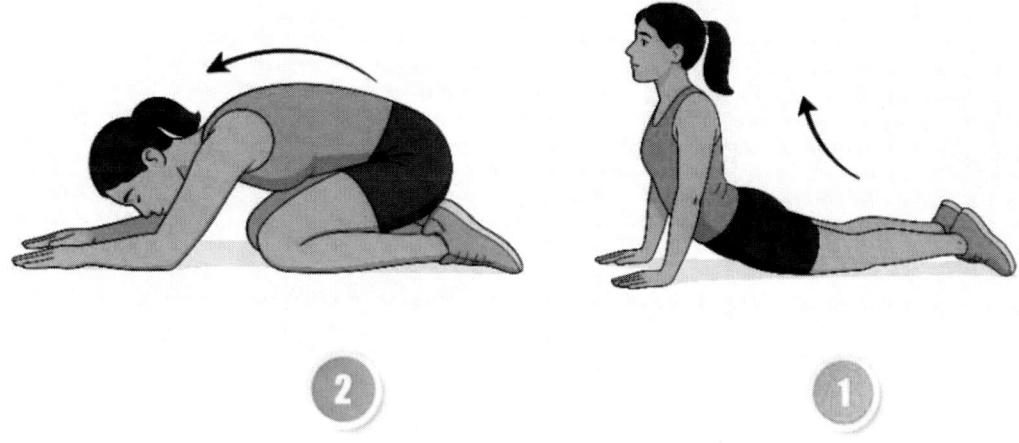

Execution Keys

- Keep **shoulders away from your ears** in both positions.
- In cobra, engage your **glutes and core** lightly to support your spine.
- Let the breath guide the transitions—**inhale to lift, exhale to fold**.
- Move smoothly, not forcefully—avoid jerky or rushed motion.

⚠ Safety Tip

If you experience lower back discomfort in cobra, reduce the height or keep your elbows bent in a "baby cobra" variation. Never lock out your arms if your lumbar spine feels compressed.

Thread-the-Needle Shoulder Stretch

Purpose

To gently stretch the shoulders, upper back, and thoracic spine—alleviating tension from pressing movements, posture strain, or prolonged sitting.

How to Perform It

1. Begin in an **all-fours position** with your hands under shoulders and knees under hips.
2. Reach your **right arm underneath your left arm**, palm facing up, and allow your right shoulder and temple to **lower to the floor**.
3. Keep your **hips stacked** over your knees and your left hand pressing gently into the mat for support.
4. Relax into the stretch and hold for **30–45 seconds**, feeling the rotation in your mid-back and shoulder.
5. Slowly return to center and **repeat on the left side**.

Execution Keys

- Let gravity do the work—don't force the reach.
- Keep your **hips still and centered**, avoiding excessive shifting.
- Soften your breathing and let your **upper body melt into the floor**.
- Press lightly through your grounded hand to control the stretch depth.

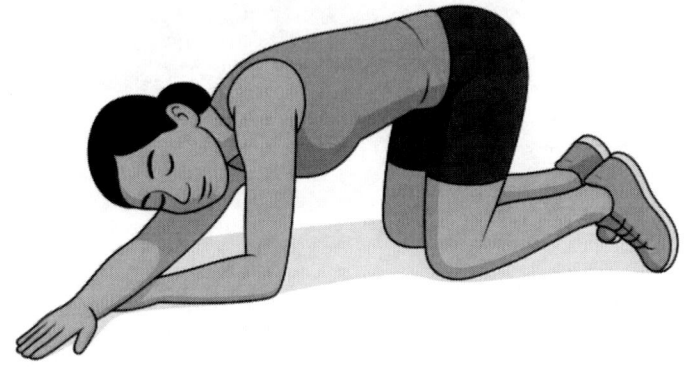

⚠ Safety Tip

Avoid this stretch if you have a recent shoulder injury or pain when rotating. Use a folded towel under your head or shoulder if full contact with the floor is uncomfortable.

Why It Matters

Thread-the-Needle targets the **posterior deltoids, traps, and thoracic spine**—areas that often accumulate tension from upper body workouts or daily posture habits. This calming pose encourages **spinal rotation, shoulder decompression**, and a parasympathetic reset that enhances mobility and reduces stiffness over time.

Chapter 9: 28-Day Bodyweight Challenge

This 28-day challenge is designed to help you build strength, improve mobility, and move with more control and confidence. It's a practical and progressive plan you can follow at home, using only your bodyweight.

You won't need any equipment or complicated routines. Each workout is simple, intentional, and structured to help you build real results. You'll begin with foundational mobility work, then progress into core training, push and pull strength, lower-body control, balance, and functional movement.

Everything you'll do here is based on the exercises already introduced earlier in the book. You're not learning anything new — you're now applying what you've already learned.

How the Challenge Works

Each day includes a short workout made up of no more than three exercises. The format is simple to follow, with clear sets, reps, and hold times. Rest days and active recovery are included to give your body time to adapt and recharge.

The focus is always on control, not speed. Your goal is to perform every movement with proper form and full attention, so you get stronger and more stable with each passing day.

What You Can Expect

By the end of this challenge, you'll likely notice real improvements in your posture, coordination, and total-body strength. Your core will feel more engaged, your joints more mobile, and your movements more balanced. You'll also build momentum — the kind that helps you stay consistent even after the challenge ends.

Take it one day at a time. Don't worry about perfection. Just show up, follow the plan, and stay present in every rep. Progress will follow.

Week 1: Foundation Phase

📖 DAY 1 — Mobility Activation

Exercise	Sets & Reps	Notes
Arm Swings	2 sets of 20	Forward & backward
Standing Hip Openers	2 sets of 10/leg	Controlled, full-range
Cat-Cow Flow	2 sets of 8 reps	Inhale on cow, exhale on cat

📖 DAY 2 — Core Stability

Exercise	Sets & Reps	Notes
Dead Bug	3 sets of 6/side	Keep lower back flat
Seated Knee Lift Hold	3 x 15 seconds	Sit tall, activate deep core
Hollow Body Hold	3 x 20 seconds	Modify by raising arms higher

📖 DAY 3 — Push Strength

Exercise	Sets & Reps	Notes
Wall Push-Ups	3 sets of 10	Focus on full range
Shoulder Taps (Wall)	3 sets of 10	Slow & stable torso
Incline Push-Ups	2 sets of 8	Keep body in straight line

📖 DAY 4 — Recovery Flow

Exercise	Sets & Reps	Notes
Hamstring Scoops	2 sets of 10/leg	Long spine, sweeping arms
Thread-the-Needle Stretch	2 x 30 sec/side	Shoulder relaxed to floor
Seated Hamstring Fold	2 x 30 sec hold	Hinge at hips, soft knees allowed

📖 DAY 5 — Lower Body Control

Exercise	Sets & Reps	Notes
Bodyweight Squats	3 sets of 12	Drive through heels
Step-Back Lunges	2 sets of 8/leg	Keep front knee over ankle
Calf Raise Hold	3 x 15 seconds	Balance at top of range

📖 DAY 6 — *Balance & Flow*

Exercise	Sets & Reps	Notes
Single-Leg Hold	2 x 20 sec/leg	Stand tall, arms by sides
Dynamic March-in-Place	2 x 30 seconds	Controlled tempo
Bear Crawl Walkout	3 sets of 4 reps	Keep knees hovering off floor

📖 DAY 7 — *Rest & Reflect*

Activity	Duration	Notes
Full Rest Day	—	No workout required
Optional: Gentle Walk	10–20 mins	Focus on posture & breathing
Optional: Breath Work	5 minutes	Inhale 4 sec, exhale 6 sec

Week 2: Strength Integration

DAY 8 — Active Mobility Reset

Exercise	Sets & Reps	Notes
Spinal Rolls	2 sets of 6 reps	Smooth and controlled
Deep Squat Hold	3 x 20 seconds	Elbows inside knees
Wrist Rolls & Pulses	2 x 10 each	Clockwise & counterclockwise

DAY 9 — Core Control

Exercise	Sets & Reps	Notes
Mountain Taps	3 sets of 10/side	Keep hips low and still
Supine Leg Slide	3 sets of 8/side	Core tight, back flat
Plank Push-Up	2 sets of 6–8 reps	Engage core, smooth transitions

DAY 10 — Pull + Push Combo

Exercise	Sets & Reps	Notes
Towel Pull	3 sets of 8–10	Squeeze shoulder blades
Doorway Row	2 sets of 6–8	Control both pull and return
Negative Push-Up	3 reps, slow lower	5-sec descent, knees if needed

📖 DAY 11 — Recovery Flow

Exercise	Sets & Reps	Notes
Reclined Twist	2 x 30 sec/side	Shoulders flat on floor
Seated Hamstring Fold	2 x 30 sec hold	Long spine, soft knees allowed
Cat-Cow Flow	2 sets of 8 reps	Inhale/exhale with spine

DAY 12 — Glutes & Isometrics

Exercise	Sets & Reps	Notes
Glute Bridge March	2 sets of 6/leg	Hips stay level
Wall Sit	2 x 30 seconds	Knees at 90°, core tight
Kneeling Hip Extension	3 sets of 8/leg	Drive heel upward, hips level

DAY 13 — Stability Challenge

Exercise	Sets & Reps	Notes
Lateral Crawl Step	3 sets of 4 steps/side	Keep knees low, hips stable
Dynamic March-in-Place	2 x 30 seconds	Slow, rhythmic, arms active
Seated Leg Extensions	2 sets of 10 reps	Upright posture, lift with control

DAY 14 — Full Rest

Activity	Duration	Notes
Full Rest Day	—	Let muscles recover fully
Optional: Breath Work	5 minutes	Inhale 4 sec, exhale 6 sec
Optional: Easy Walking	10–20 minutes	Gentle pace, relaxed focus

Week 3: Progress & Precision

DAY 15 — Mobility Reset + Flow

Exercise	Sets & Reps	Notes
Standing Hip Openers	2 sets of 10/leg	Smooth circles, upright posture
Leg Swings (front-back)	2 sets of 10/leg	Controlled arc, hold wall if needed
Spinal Rolls	2 sets of 6 reps	Roll up slowly from the hips

DAY 16 — Core Stability Progression

Exercise	Sets & Reps	Notes
Lying Windshield Wipers	3 sets of 6/side	Keep upper back grounded
Seated Leg Extensions	3 sets of 10 reps	Engage hip flexors and core
Reverse Tabletop Hold	2 × 20 seconds	Squeeze glutes and lift chest

DAY 17 — Pull Strength Progression

Exercise	Sets & Reps	Notes
Wall Pull-Backs	3 sets of 10 reps	Hands slide along wall
Reverse Arm Flaps	3 x 30 seconds	Squeeze shoulder blades together
Dead Hang (if possible)	2 × 10–20 seconds	Optional: if equipment available

📖 DAY 18 — Recovery Day

Exercise	Sets & Reps	Notes
Reclined Twist	2 × 30 sec/side	Keep both shoulders flat
Seated Hamstring Fold	2 × 30 sec hold	Fold from hips, not spine
Thread-the-Needle Stretch	2 × 30 sec/side	Relax into the shoulder

DAY 19 — Lower Body Strength & Balance

Exercise	Sets & Reps	Notes
Supported Pistol Prep	3 sets of 5/leg	Use chair/pole for support
Calf Raise Hold	3 × 15 seconds	Rise as tall as possible
Chair Sit-Down/Stand-Up	2 sets of 10 reps	Control the descent

DAY 20 — Flow + Coordination

Exercise	Sets & Reps	Notes
Wall-Assisted Handstand Hold	3 × 10–20 sec	Engage core and press through shoulders
Dynamic March-in-Place	3 × 30 seconds	High knees, arms opposite
Bear Crawl Walkout	3 sets of 4 reps	Keep back flat, knees hover

DAY 21 — Rest Day

Activity	Duration	Notes
Full Rest	—	No formal training
Optional: Gentle Mobility	10 minutes	Choose favorites from Days 1, 4, or 8
Optional: Light Breathing	5 minutes	Inhale 4 sec, exhale 6 sec

Week 4: Control, Flow & Integration

DAY 22 — Mobility Reset & Flow

Exercise	Sets & Reps	Notes
Wrist Rolls & Pulses	2 x 10 each way	Loosen up wrists, full circles
Hamstring Scoops	2 x 10 per leg	Straight legs, reach and sweep
Deep Squat Hold	2 x 30 seconds	Elbows inside knees, chest up

📖 DAY 23 — Core Integration

Exercise	Sets & Reps	Notes
Bird Dog Reach	3 sets of 6/side	Opposite limbs, keep spine stable
Plank Push-Up	2 sets of 8 reps	Slow, strong transitions
Hollow Body Hold	3 × 20 seconds	Low back stays in contact

📖 DAY 24 — Controlled Push + Pull

Exercise	Sets & Reps	Notes
Incline Push-Ups	3 sets of 10 reps	Use bench, keep straight line
Doorway Row	3 sets of 6–8 reps	Slow pull, squeeze upper back
Wall Slides	2 sets of 10 reps	Elbows, wrists glide along wall

📖 DAY 25 — Active Recovery Flow

Exercise	Sets & Reps	Notes
Seated Hamstring Fold	2 x 30 sec hold	Flex feet, reach gently
Cobra to Child's Pose Flow	3 sets of 4 flows	Breathe slowly through each
Standing Forward Fold	2 x 30 sec hold	Knees soft, head heavy

DAY 26 — Lower Body Balance + Control

Exercise	Sets & Reps	Notes
Single-Leg Reach	3 sets of 6/leg	Hinge at hips, stay stable
Step-Back Lunges	2 sets of 8/leg	Controlled depth, upright torso
Chair Sit-Down/Stand-Up	2 sets of 10 reps	No hands, slow tempo

DAY 27 — Flow Integration & Recovery

Exercise	Sets & Reps	Notes
Thread-the-Needle Stretch	2 x 30 sec/side	Relax shoulder into floor
Cobra to Child's Pose Flow	2 sets of 4 flows	Focus on smooth transition
Kneeling Hip Flexor Stretch	2 x 30 sec/side	Squeeze glute to deepen stretch

DAY 28 — Final Rest + Reflection

Activity	Duration	Notes
Full Rest	—	No physical work, just reflection
Optional: Gentle Walk	10–20 minutes	Breathe deeply and enjoy movement
Optional: Write Reflections	—	What improved? What's next?

Conclusion

You've reached the end of this foundational guide to calisthenics—but your personal journey is just beginning.

Over the past chapters, you've explored the building blocks of bodyweight training—from mobility and core stability to push-pull mechanics, balance, and total-body control. You've learned that progress in calisthenics isn't about gimmicks or perfection—it's about mastery of form, consistency, and mindful progression. Every rep, every set, every pause in discomfort—these moments build not just your body, but your discipline and confidence.

The 28-Day Challenge gave you structure. Now it's time to build your own. Return to these exercises with greater intensity, longer holds, or added variations. Mix routines based on what your body needs most—mobility one day, strength the next. Use your own progress as the benchmark.

Remember:

- You don't need a gym to grow stronger.
- You don't need perfect conditions to train.
- You just need your body, your breath, and your commitment.

Keep showing up. Some days will be tough. Some days, your best effort might just be a deep breath and a light stretch. That's okay. Growth honors the effort, not just the outcome.

THANK YOU

Made in United States
North Haven, CT
25 October 2025

81391640R00052